EXERCISES FOR

MULTIPLE SCLEROSIS

A Safe and Effective Program to Fight Fatigue, Build Strength, and Improve Balance

Brad Hamler

Foreword by Ben W. Thrower, M.D.

Contributions by Matt Bloom

Photography by Peter Field Peck

healthyliving**books**

New York • London

A HEALTHY LIVING BOOK
Published by
Hatherleigh Press
5-22 46th Avenue, Suite 200
Long Island City, NY 11101
www.healthylivingbooks.com

Library of Congress Cataloging-in-Publication Data

Hamler, Brad.
  Exercises for multiple sclerosis : a safe and effective program to fight
fatigue, build strength, and improve balance / by Brad Hamler ;
contributions by Matt Bloom ; foreword by Ben W. Thrower ; photography by
Peter Field Peck.
     p. cm.
  ISBN 1-57826-227-5
  1. Multiple sclerosis--Popular works. 2. Multiple
sclerosis--Treatment--Popular works. 3. Exercise--Popular works. 4.
Self-care, Health. I. Title.
  RC377.H36 2006
  616.8'34062--dc22
                          2006017939

All forms of exercise pose some inherent risks. The information in this book is meant to supple-
ment, not replace, proper exercise training. Before practicing the exercises in this book, be sure that
your equipment is well maintained. Do not take risks beyond your level of experience, training,
and fitness. The exercise programs are not intended as a substitute for any exercise routine or treatment that may have been prescribed by your doctor. As with all exercise programs, you should get
your doctor's approval before beginning. The authors(s), editors, and publisher advise readers to
take full responsibility for their safety and know their limits.

Healthy Living Books are available for bulk purchase, special promotions, and premiums. For
information on reselling and special purchase opportunities, please call us at 1-800-528-2550 and
ask for the Special Sales Manager.

Cover and interior design by Deborah Miller and Jacinta Monniere
Thanks to the models: Elizabeth Dykes and Peter DeFresco

10 9 8 7 6 5 4 3 2
Printed in Canada

Dedication

This book is dedicated to all of my clients who are fighting multiple sclerosis (MS) with determination and courage. It was because you were open to the possibilities that made my work and this book happen. It has been my honor and privilege to share it with you. Thank you!

Acknowledgments

To Hatherleigh, for doing a third book with me. Thank you to Andrea Au, Alyssa Smith, and Kevin Moran for your patience during the writing process. To Dr. Ben Thrower, for your unique style and approach that seemed to fit my unconventional ways. To the staff of the MS Center at Shepherd in Atlanta, Georgia, especially Tracy Walker. To the National MS Society (Atlanta Chapter), Director Roy Rangel and coordinator Christine John for your belief in me; my daughter Katja: you are my inspiration; and to Millie, my wife: thank you for hanging in there with me through it all.

In memory of a good friend, Jim Brousquet.

Table of Contents

Foreword

Every week, 200 people in the United States are given the news that they have multiple sclerosis (MS). For some, this is a big shock. Others have dealt with symptoms for years and almost welcome an explanation to their mystery. Information regarding MS is readily available; some good and some not so good. One of my favorite patients remembers sitting in the exam room after we had the "you have MS" discussion. He says all he could think was, "Multiple sclerosis... multiple sclerosis... who did I sleep with that has multiple sclerosis?!" (Note for the uninitiated: MS is not a sexually transmitted disease.)

As a neurologist, I only work with MS. I cannot think of a more challenging and rewarding group of people to care for. The MS community is incredibly diverse, but they do share some common traits. Inquisitive, adaptable, Internet savvy—all are terms that apply to many people with MS. Combine these traits with the complex and variable nature of the disease itself, and it is little wonder that a comprehensive wellness approach works best in dealing with MS.

The past few years have seen a rapid advance in our understanding of how MS works and what we can do about it. Some discoveries also serve to humble us as to the complexities of our human bodies. Major research focuses upon finding the best possible option to stop MS progression, how to understand the genetic and environmental factors that lead to MS, and repairing the damage done so that function might be restored.

So where does exercise fit in this MS picture? It wasn't so long ago that people with MS were told not to exercise. The fear was that fatigue would be worsened or that new symptoms could be provoked with exercise. What a difference twenty years makes! We now know that exercise is not only tolerated in MS, but it may be beneficial in a number of ways.

Studies have shown that exercise does not reduce relapse rates or slow progression of disability. Regular exercise can make a difference, though, in how a person with MS feels and functions. Exercise can improve fatigue in MS. This alone should impact a person's quality of life, especially since fatigue is listed on most MS patient's worst complaint list. Improvements in walking and lung function have also been noted.

It's human nature to want a quick fix for our problems. People with MS are no different. Modern medicine offers more hope now than ever for the MS community. However, medications cannot provide all of the answers to wellness. Exercise and nutrition should complement medical therapy. The person with MS faces the same challenges in sticking with an exercise regimen as anyone else, and then some. Some days it's just so tempting to sleep in. Many MS symptoms pose additional hurdles to starting and maintaining exercise. And then there's the variable nature of the symptoms themselves. "Which body am I going to wake up in today?" you may wonder.

I have seen the benefits of a dedicated personal trainer's attention to my MS patients. The author, Brad Hamler, came to my attention through the work he was doing with the MS community. Several of my patients raved about the benefits they were seeing through training with Brad. I can remember one lady coming in for a follow-up visit at the Shepherd Center. She had an extra bounce in her step and just looked, well… well. In my mind, I was sure that it must be due to a medication that we had started, stopped, increased, decreased, or in some other way manipulated. "Come, behold the wonders of my medical prowess!" I humbly thought. But no, she was doing better because of the regular exercise regimen she was doing with Brad.

Finding a personal trainer who is knowledgeable in regards to MS is always a blessing. Finding one with that spark of extra commitment is rare. Brad is one of those folks. He has gone above and beyond by helping with educational programs and MS non-profit fundraisers. Some things you learn in books, some you learn through experience. Through this book, you can take advantage of Brad's exercise knowledge, gained through both sources.

People don't choose to have MS. They don't choose the course that their MS will take. But we can all choose to be as fit as our bodies will allow. If you have MS, this book will be your guide to getting fit safely.

Good luck to you! Now get going!

Ben W. Thrower, M.D.
Medical Director of the Multiple Sclerosis Center
at the Shepherd Center

Introduction

Maintenance Is Progress

When I first presented my theory Maintenance is Progress (MIP) in *Beginners Luck* (Hatherleigh Press), it was to help the beginner learn the basics of exercise necessary for an effective workout. The premise of Maintenance is Progress is: "Learn to train safely, effectively, and consistently—for a lifetime." This should be the motto for this book as well. While maintenance literally means "to stay the same", exercise maintenance needs to be progressive in order to work.

By using MIP, you can make exercise part of your daily life and end the cycle of overtraining. Remember, it's not advisable for anyone to go into a gym and attempt too much too soon. This type of overtraining will cause unnecessary soreness, and often leads new exercisers to quit—a common scenario that is absolutely avoidable by instead following MIP. MIP is also useful to help avoid the pitfalls of inconsistent training (yo-yo exercising). This is the practice of working out consistently for a number of weeks and then stopping, or even working out so hard that you potentially injure yourself or become frustrated with the lack of instant results.

In my second book, *Extreme Training* (Hatherleigh Press), I applied the ideals of MIP to the fitness enthusiast. In long term fitness, it becomes even more important to understand Maintenance really is Progress. Over the years, the amount of visible progress from training becomes much less (the basic law of diminishing returns). MIP may slow down the aging process, because by learning to exercise in a safe and effective manner, you are creating a progressive fitness program that is easily maintained.

Maintenance is Progress can also be used by those with MS. When my clients learned how to train safely and effectively, they were able to stay stronger and more functional. Their workouts gave them the additional strength they needed to help fight the disease. With MS, working out with maximum efficiency is vital! You want to receive the most benefits from exercise possible before your fatigue becomes a factor.

My clients began training with this mindset and soon started reporting results. My clients experienced fewer or more manageable effects from MS—it was described as taking much less of a toll on their bodies. I began to observe changes in my clients as well—they carried themselves with new confidence. This experimental physical fitness regimen convinced me that more evidence is needed to find out the connection between improved fitness and lowered fatigue.

When I was working with Dr. Ben Thrower's patients, I had yet another opportunity to watch how Maintenance is Progress helped in the fight against MS. When his patients went in for their annual MRI scan, those who were also training with me showed no new lesions forming at several sites on the scans. It was exciting and rewarding to see their hard work pay off.

One thing I did notice was that the more consistently a client trained, the easier their ability to maintain their progress. As you go through this book, remember what I've said here. I hope you take Maintenance is Progress to heart and start on your own path to controlling MS and your own body.

Part I: About Multiple Sclerosis

1

What Is Multiple Sclerosis?

Multiple sclerosis (MS) affects not only those with it, but also their family members, friends, physicians, medical staff, and counselors. Its unpredictability makes it a particularly challenging disease. Yet although the causes of and cure for MS are still being investigated, the good news is that MS can be managed with the proper diet and exercise.

MS most commonly starts between the ages of 20 and 40. It affects women almost twice as much as it does men, and whites almost twice as much as it does other races. Although not an inherited disease, susceptibility to MS does run in families. Environmental factors influencing the onset of MS are being closely studied. For example, MS is much more prevalent in temperate climates than in the tropics. The theory that MS could be the result of a virus or viruses is supported by evidence that MS spreads with the movement from place to place of those suffering from it.

Once diagnosed with MS, you may feel frightened and alone. You may feel angry at your doctors and at your own helplessness. To make things more difficult, your family and friends might be looking to you for answers and reassurance. Perhaps the worst thing is being perceived differently, receiving sympathy without true empathy. And you now have a new identity: MS Patient.

It's important to know that there are many misconceptions about MS. Perhaps the most common one is that MS is fatal. This isn't true at all. Statistics show that most people with MS have almost normal life spans. Another misperception is that all MS sufferers end up in wheelchairs. The truth is that after twenty years of untreated MS, ⅔ of people are not in wheelchairs. Because there is no cure for MS, many believe nothing can be done for it. This, once again, isn't true. Exercise is one significant thing that can be done, as will be detailed in this book. Having MS in no way means you can't live a full life, spiritually, emotionally, and sexually. And the contention that scientists are not making much progress against MS is absolutely untrue. No medicines were available to counter the disease until 1993. Now there are five approved drugs for the various forms of MS. The National MS Society now spends $30 million annually to fund three hundred studies on all aspects of the disease.

If you or someone you know has multiple sclerosis, it's important to understand what the disease is and how it impacts the body. Briefly, multiple sclerosis is an inflammatory disease affecting the central nervous system (CNS), which is the brain and the spinal cord. MS causes plaques or lesions to appear on areas of the brain known as "white matter," the nerve fibers (neurons) that transmit signals within the CNS and between the CNS and the peripheral nervous system (PNS), which consists of the nerves that serve the rest of the body.

A closer look at these lesions reveals that myelin, or the protective fatty protein that sheathes and insulates the nerve, has been worn away in a process called demyelination. Demyelination occurs during periods called relapses and results in nerve messages being sent from the CNS to the rest of the body more slowly and less efficiently. In 1998, it was discovered that MS also damages the nerve fibers, axons, themselves. This type of damage results in more permanent symptoms. The scar tissue that then forms over the affected area during remission periods, a process called remyelination, can further hinder brain and spinal cord communication with the rest of the body.

Strong evidence suggests that MS is an autoimmune disease. This means that the T cell, a type of white blood cell responsible for identifying and destroying harmful invaders, mistakenly identifies parts of the body's own tissue as harmful and attacks it. In the case of MS, T cells attack the myelin sheathes protecting the nerves of the CNS. This causes the plaques and lesions described above, as well as symptoms that will be discussed later.

Types of Multiple Sclerosis

Although MS is an unpredictable disease, one certainty is that your MS will take a different course than anyone else's. That said, the disease usually follows a general pattern. For example, inflammation of the CNS in the early stages of the disease doesn't produce any symptoms, so no one, including the person with MS, is aware that there is anything wrong. Some researchers believe that 40 percent of people with MS have this type, and only autopsies reveal that they ever had MS. Only after the disease progresses do the inflammatory lesions start to produce symptoms. As it continues to progress, remissions from the symptom-producing relapses become less complete and leave residual effects. Further progression produces worse symptoms, and disability becomes more severe. In the worst cases, symptoms not only worsen but persist without abating. The progression just described has been categorized into four main types of MS.

Relapsing/Remitting MS (RRMS)

Relapses or exacerbations are the dominant feature of this type of MS. During relapses, which can last from only days to as long as months, new symptoms can appear and old ones can re-emerge or worsen. Myelin is damaged during relapses, and this causes inflammation and lesions. Periods of remission follow relapses. This means that inflammation subsides and cells called oligodendrocytes repair the myelin (remyelination). During remissions, the victim recovers either fully or partially, a process that can be slow and gradual or almost instantaneous. Most people with MS have this type, and it is typically acquired while in their twenties or thirties. Twice as many women as men have RRMS.

Secondary Progressive MS (SPMS)

This is the phase of MS that follows relapsing/remitting MS. The disease worsens between relapses, and relapses become longer until they merge into a general progression. Apart from a few brief remissions following relapses, there is no real recovery. Fifty percent of people with relapsing/remitting MS develop secondary progressive (SPMS) after ten years. The figure rises to 95 percent after twenty-five to thirty years.

Primary Progressive MS (PPMS)

In this type of MS, the disease progresses steadily with no remissions at all except for an occasional leveling off of symptoms. Men get this type of MS as often as women do, and onset usually occurs in the late thirties and early forties. PPMS often spreads to the brain but is less likely to damage the brain than PPMS or SPMS is. This means that people with PPMS are less likely to suffer from cognitive problems.

Other Types of MS and Diseases Similar to MS

Benign MS

This describes MS in people who have had it for fifteen or more years without suffering any serious disabilities.

Malignant MS

This rare type of MS is also called Marburg's variant or acute multiple sclerosis. It progresses rapidly from onset and causes severe disability.

Transitional/ Progressive MS

This type of MS is no longer referred to very much, but it progresses steadily years after an isolated bout.

Devic's Disease

Also called neuromyelitis optica, this disease is related to MS and it attacks nerves in the eyes and the spinal cord. A recently developed antibody test allows for the accurate diagnosis of this demyelinating disorder.

Balo's Concentric Sclerosis

Although very similar to MS, Balo's lesions form in rings of intact myelin and demyelinated zones.

What Causes MS and Who is Affected by It?

Now that you have a basic understanding of what MS is and its various types, you're probably wondering who gets it, how they get it, and what causes it. Although nothing definitive has been discovered, doctors and scientists have noticed certain patterns and factors that are leading them toward answers to these questions.

Age

MS rarely begins before the age of 15 or after the age of 60.

Race

Whites are more than twice as likely to get MS as blacks.

Gender

Due to the different biochemistry of their bodies, MS affects almost twice as many women than men. Estrogen and progesterone, found in women, have an immunomodulating function that may influence the onset and course of the disease. Women also have a different genetic makeup than men. They possess two X chromosomes while men possess one X and one Y chromosome. If it is true that genes play a role in the onset of MS, then it is possible that the X gene may play a particular role.

Geography

MS strikes most often in temperate latitudes and in the western hemisphere, specifically in Europe, North America, Australia and New Zealand. Regions north of 40 degrees latitude have a much higher incidence than regions south of that latitude. And although MS is found in Japan and China, it occurs much more rarely in those countries. The reason for the discrepancy between the incidences of MS in northern and southern parts of the world is still largely unknown, although recent research suggests that it may have to do with the seasonal fluctuations of sunlight in temperate climates that affects body chemistry. Studies supporting this show that onset and remission of MS are more common in springtime and least common during the winter. This may be due to the levels of vitamin D3, melatonin and other biochemicals, which vary along with the seasons.

Genetics

The connection between the incidence of MS and genetics is in many ways more convincing than the connection between MS and geography. This is because the similarity between temperate regions in the Western Hemisphere, where MS is much more common, and temperate regions in the Eastern Hemisphere, where it is rare, are greater than the similarities between these regions and the tropics.

And although it is commonly accepted that genes play a major role in the onset of MS, the particular genes responsible for the disease remain unidentified. To make matters more complicated, scientists suspect that genes working in tandem as opposed to individual genes, and combinations of genes working in tandem with other gene combinations, might result in a predisposition for MS.

Allergic Reaction

Although not yet widely supported, some believe that MS can be caused by an allergic reaction. They prescribe histamines as a treatment.

Childbirth

It follows that if female hormones heighten the risk of developing MS, then pregnancy and the hormonal changes it brings may affect the disease. Studies show that it does, initially in a positive rather than a negative manner. Pregnant women have a significantly lower rate of relapse. But while the rate of relapse during pregnancy generally declines, it increases significantly three months after birth before falling back to prepregnancy levels.

Diet

Studies show that countries with diets high in the saturated fats found in dairy and meat products have a much higher incidence of MS. Conversely, people in countries such as Japan who eat very little saturated fat and a lot of fish, soy, and seeds have much lower incidences. This leads researchers to believe that the essential fatty acid deficiency that results from excessive consumption of saturated fats might contribute to development of multiple sclerosis.

Viral Infection

The fact that most MS patients have high levels of antibodies to measles and other viruses suggests that MS might be the body's delayed reaction to these viruses.

Conclusion

As you can see, the medical community and researchers do not yet know what really causes MS. There as many theories as there are ways this disease emerges. This can be very discouraging. What I've experienced is that my clients do not care as much about what causes MS as much as not allowing the disease to dictate their quality of life postdiagnosis.

Over the years I have been asked by the National Multiple Sclerosis Society to speak at its functions. I usually speak directly after a doctor who speaks on "What Is MS?" The physician speaks at length about the mind-numbing details of this disease. I watch the faces of the attendees, and their attention drifts almost immediately. It's just too much, even when there is a definite need for a neurologist to cover this material. Dr. Ben Thrower is an exceptional speaker, and it is not a mere coincidence that he and I are presenting *Exercises for Multiple Sclerosis* together. He has a unique ability to keep audiences engaged as well as informed.

By the time it is my turn to speak, the room of MS patients seems as if they have been hit over the head repeatedly—their energy is down. The first thing I get everyone to do is to stand up and raise their arms over their heads. I have them repeat this motion more than once, and they begin to moan and groan. I finally tell them to sit and remain in their chairs, to which the response is a collective sigh. It is at this moment I say, "Good job! You have all just finished your first exercise." The response is always laughter and a feeling of accomplishment. This is when I say, "No one in this room is disabled!"

I'm not going to tell you that you can be cured of MS by exercising. However, you can be enabled in a different way by an act of will and proper motivation. Learn how to begin this process of creating exercises for your body, because no matter where you are now, you can change the quality of your life.

2

Diagnosing Multiple Sclerosis

Diagnosing multiple sclerosis is the first step toward treating it. However, because MS attacks the central nervous system (CNS), which controls almost all bodily functions, its symptoms vary widely. Additionally, only a few symptoms of MS are unique to the disease, so having more than one of them doesn't mean you have MS. Almost no one with MS will have all of the various symptoms listed below. This makes diagnosis even more difficult. Nonetheless, doctors use these symptoms as clues for your diagnosis.

The Most Common Symptoms

The first indicators that you might have multiple sclerosis are the various symptoms it produces. Mental and physical fatigue and spasticity are the most common MS symptoms, and the majority of people with MS will experience one or all of them, often chronically.

Mental Fatigue

Mental fatigue can be mild or severe, and it is usually made worse by overexertion and increased body or environmental temperature. Its intensity usually fluctuates during the course of the day: Sufferers often feel fine in the morning but worn down by afternoon. A nap can help you recover.

Physical Fatigue

Physical fatigue can result from as little as a short walk. This is a result of the reduced efficiency of the nerves caused by demyelination. Rest usually helps, but recovery times vary according to how far the disease has progressed. A hot environment makes both mental and physical fatigue worse.

Spasticity

Spasticity is involuntary muscle contractions that are not coordinated with the other muscles. To explain further, most muscles in the human body, such as the biceps and triceps, are paired and work opposing each other. When the bicep contracts, the triceps is stretched, thus bending the arm. When the triceps contracts, the bicep stretches, thus extending the arm. In order for this to happen, signals have to be sent from the CNS through a network of peripheral nerves, which then relay sensory information, such as heat, cold, and pain, back to the CNS. MS can impair the balance between muscles that flex and muscles that contract. This usually results in too much extensor muscle tone in the legs and too much flexion in the arms. This chronic state of too much muscle tone is called spasticity. When it comes in a sudden wave of cramping, it's called a spasm.

Spasticity can be painful, and it manifests in an uncoordinated gait, stiff posture, and restricted range of limb movement. Muscles can be permanently shortened (contracture), and the joints that muscles affected by spasticity are attached to can be damaged. However, one benefit of spasticity is that reflexive spasms of the muscles increases their tone, which reduces atrophy.

Other Symptoms

The following is a list of other MS symptoms.

Visual

Optic neuritis: Blurred vision, eye pain, loss of color vision, blindness.

Diplopia: Double vision

Nystagmus: Jerky eye movements

Ocular dymetria: Constant under- or overshooting eye movements.

Internuclear ophthalmoplegia: Lack of coordination between the two eyes, nystagmus, diplopia.

Movement and sound phosphenes: Seeing flashing lights when moving eyes or in response to a sudden noise.

Afferent pupillary defect: Abnormal pupil responses.

Motor

Paresis, monoparesis, paraparesis, hemiparesis, quadriparesis: Muscle weakness: partial or mild paralysis

Plegia, paraplegia, hemiplegia, tetraplegia, quadriplegia: Paralysis: total or near-total loss of muscle strength

Dysarthria: Slurred speech and related speech problems.

Muscle atrophy: Wasting of muscles due to lack of use.

Spasms, cramps: Involuntary contraction of muscles

Hypotonia, clonus: Problems with posture.

Myoclonus, myokymia: Jerking and twitching muscles, Tics.

Restless leg syndrome: Involuntary leg movements, especially bothersome at night.

Footdrop: Foot drags along floor during walking.

Dysfunctional reflexes: MSRs, Babinski's, Hoffmann's, Chaddock's.

Sensory

Paraesthesia: Partial numbness, tingling, buzzing and vibration sensations.

Anaesthesia: Complete numbness/loss of sensation.

Neuralgia; neuropathic and neurogenic pain: Pain without apparent cause, burning, itching and electrical shock sensations.

Lhermitte's sign: Electric shocks and buzzing sensations when moving head.

Proprioceptive dysfunction: Loss of awareness of location of body parts.

Trigeminal neuralgia: Facial pain.

Coordination and Balance

Ataxia: Loss of coordination.

Intention tremor: Shaking when performing fine movements.

Dysmetria: Constant under- or overshooting limb movements.

Vestibular ataxia: Abnormal balance function in the inner ear.

Vertigo: Nausea/vomiting/sensitivity to travel sickness from vestibular ataxia.

Speech ataxia: Problems coordinating speech, stuttering.

Dystonia: Slow limb position feedback.

Dysdiadochokinesia: Loss of ability to produce rapidly alternating movements. Example: inability to move to a rhythm.

Bowel, Bladder, and Sexual Symptoms

Frequent micturation, bladder spasticity: Urinary urgency and incontinence.

Flaccid bladder, detrusor-sphincter dyssynergia: Urinary hesitancy and retention.

Erectile dysfunction: Male and female impotence.

Anorgasmy: Inability to achieve orgasm.

Retrograde ejaculation: Ejaculating into the bladder.

Frigidity: Inability to become sexually aroused.

Constipation: Infrequent or irregular bowel movements.

Fecal urgency: Bowel urgency.

Fecal incontinence: Bowel incontinence.

Cognitive

Depression: Depressed mood.

Cognitive dysfunction: Short-term and long-term memory problems, forgetfulness, slow word recall.

Dementia: Loss of intellectual functions.

Mood swings, emotional liability, euphoria.

Bipolar syndrome: Formerly known as manic depression.

Anxiety.

Aphasia, dysphasia: Impairments to speech comprehension and production.

Other

Uhthoff's symptom: Increase in severity of symptoms with heat.

Gastroesophageal reflux: Acid reflux, impaired sense of taste and smell, epileptic seizures, swallowing problems, respiratory problems.

Sleep disorders.

Inappropriately cold body parts.

Autonomic nervous system problems.

Complications

In advanced cases of MS, you are confined to a bed or chair. This can lead to complications such as urinary tract infections, skin ulcers, pneumonia, pulmonary embolisms (blood clots in the lungs), and various side effects from prescribed drugs.

Diagnosing Multiple Sclerosis

One reason why diagnosing multiple sclerosis is so difficult is because there is no single test for it. Researchers are still unsure if MS is just one disease or a combination of them. The process of diagnosis therefore involves elimination of many other possibilities, which can take a long time and is often frustrating for the one suffering those symptoms. The following are some but certainly not all of the diseases commonly tested for to determine if someone has MS:

Diseases Investigated Before Tested For MS

- Tumor or other spinal cord compression
- Stroke
- Acute disseminated encephalomyletis (ADEM)
- Lyme Disease
- Subacute sclerosing panencephalitis
- Neurosyphilis
- Progressive multifocal leukoencephalopathy
- Systemic lupus erythematosus
- Cerebral arteritis
- Complicated migraine
- Diabetes
- Hypothyroidism
- Myasthenia gravis
- Acute transverse myelitis
- Herpes simplex
- Encephalitis
- Polyarteritis nodusa
- Sjorgen syndrome
- Behcet's syndrome
- Sarcoidosis
- Paraneoplastic syndromes
- Neuromyelitis optica (Devic's syndrome)
- HIV-associated myelopathy
- Adrenomyeloneuropathy
- Myelopathy
- Spinocerebellar syndromes
- Hereditary spastic paraparesis
- Guillain-Barre syndrome
- Polymyositis
- Benign paroxysmal positional vertigo

- Parkinson's disease
- Cerebral hemorrhage
- Amyotrophic lateral sclerosis (ALS)
- Mononeuritis
- Huntington's disease
- Postinfectious encephalitis
- Arteriovenous malformations
- Arachnoid cysts
- Arnold-Chiari malformations
- Cervical spondylosis

Once all the above diseases have been eliminated, tests will be performed based on the neurological symptoms that exist. The following are some of the more common tests used to determine if a person has MS:

Romberg's sign: This is a test for ataxia, which is lack of coordination and/or clumsiness that is not caused by muscular weakness. The test requires the patient to stand with his feet together and his eyes closed, a difficult task for someone with ataxia.

Gait and coordination: Ataxia is tested for by having the patient walk normally, than heel-to-toe, and by performing finger-to-nose tests. Neurologists also look for tremors while the patient performs small motor movements.

Heel/shin test: This test for ataxia and cerebellar dysfunction is done by the patient bringing the ball of his heel onto the knee of his other leg, then moving his foot down his shin.

Lhermitte's sign: To test for lesions on the spinal cord, the patient lowers his head towards his chest. Buzzing, tingling, or electrical shocks will result if the patient is Lhermitte's positive.

Optic neuritis: This test requires the patient to read letters on a board and it determines color vision by using an Ishihara color chart.

Hearing loss: The neurologist clicks his fingers beside the patient's ear and asks him which ear the click was done next to.

Muscle strength: Various muscle groups are tested for their ability to resist pressure by the neurologist. Asymmetrical weakness is easier to determine than symmetrical weakness.

Reflexes: A rubber-coated hammer is tapped against the kneecap to measure reflexes, which can be normal, too brisk, or nonexistent.

Babinski's sign: This is a test for disease in the motor neurons of the pyramidal tract. A semisharp object is drawn along the bottom of the foot. The toes flexing downward is the normal response. In babies and people with neurological problems of the corticospinal tract, the big toe points upward.

Chaddock's sign: The skin on the outside of the patient's ankle is touched in order to test for lesions in the corticospinal tract. An upward fanning of the big toe is a positive response.

Hoffman's sign: This is another test for problems of the corticospinal tract. The nail of the third or fourth finger is tapped. Flexing of the terminal phalanx of the thumb is a positive response.

Doll's eye sign: The neurologist is looking for dissociation between the eyes and the head. The eyes moving up while the head moves down are a positive indicator.

Sensory loss: Tuning forks and pins are used to test sensory perception levels in various parts of the body.

It should be noted that a definite diagnosis of MS is almost never based entirely upon these tests. Most neurologists would next have the patient undergo further tests, such as magnetic resonance imagining (MRI).

Further Tests for MS

Newer techniques are giving additional insights beyond those of traditional MRI. For now, these are not part of routine MS management.

Magnetic Resonance Imaging

MRI is by far the most definitive diagnostic tool available to neurologists. First used in 1977, it detects abnormalities inside soft body tissue. Water molecules in the body emit small electromagnetic waves that make them act like tiny magnets. The powerful magnetic field the MRI exerts around the patient causes the water molecules in his body to wobble. The MRI, often with the help of a contrasting agent called gadolinium, detects and prints the detailed images of the brain and spinal cord formed by this wobble. MS lesions show up as paler areas in these images. Despite its capabilities, the MRI is rarely used alone to diagnose MS. The clinical and neurological tests described earlier almost always accompany it. Traditionally, MS has been defined by the presence of two clinical attacks separated by time and space. The McDonald Criteria of 2001 allow for a diagnosis of MS in a person with only one attack, if the MRI shows new lesions developing.

Functional MRI (fMRI)

fMRI uses radio waves and a strong magnetic field to measure the correlation between physical changes in the brain, such as blood flow, and mental functioning during performance of cognitive tasks.

Magnetic Resonance Spectroscopy (MRS)

MRS provides information about the brain's biochemistry, particularly the level of *N*-acetyl aspartate. Low levels of this chemical can cause nerve damage.

Magnetization Transfer Imaging (MTI)

By calculating the amount of "free water" in white matter tissue, MTI can detect abnormalities before they are detected by standard

MRI. Demyelinated and damaged nerves display higher levels of "free" than "bound" water particles.

Diffusion-Tensor Magnetic Imaging (DT-MRI or DTI)

DT-MRI causes constantly-in-motion water molecules to spread out. This diffusion is mapped and three-dimensional images of the brain are produced showing the size and location of demyelinated portions. Changes can then be measured against the progression of the disease.

Spinal Tap

Spinal tap, also called lumbar puncture, is the sampling of cerebrospinal fluid taken from close to the spinal cord. Cerebrospinal fluid surrounds the CNS and serves as a shock absorber, carrier of nutrition, waste disposer, and transmitter of messages. In this test, blood is also taken from the arm and some of the blood serum is isolated. The cerebrospinal fluid and the blood serum then undergo a procedure called electrophoresis, in which molecules in both are separated by size and electrical charge. The procedure identifies and differentiates proteins, which helps doctors diagnosis MS. 95 percent of people with MS have oligoclonal bands, which means they have a higher level of an antibody protein called immunoglobin-G in their cerebrospinal fluid than in their blood serum.

Evoked Potential (EP) Tests

Evoked potential tests measure the speed of impulses along neurons. Responses are measured by electrodes attached to the scalp and other areas of the skin. The response times in MS patients are then measured against response times for people without MS. The findings are significant because demyelinated neurons transmit signals more slowly than myelinated neurons do. Because remyelinated neurons also transmit signals more slowly, this test allows neurologists to detect older lesions. There are three types of EP tests:

Visually Evoked Potential (VEP): This test measures the speed of the optic nerve by having the patient focus on a TV screen on which there is a black-and-white-checkered pattern. The patient covers one eye, then the other. Eighty-five to 90 percent of people with definite MS and 58 percent of people with probable MS have abnormal VEP test results.

Brainstem Auditory Evoked Response (BAER): This test measures the speed of impulses along the auditory part of cranial nerve VIII, which is located in the Pons area of the brainstem. For this reason, the test may indicate lesions on the brainstem. Sixty-seven percent of people with definite MS and 41 percent of people with probable MS have abnormal BAER test results.

Somatosensory Evoked Potential (SSEP): An electrical stimulus is strapped around an arm or leg, and the current is switched on for five seconds. Electrodes attached to the back and skull measure the response in various areas. This helps neurologists determine the extent of demyelination. Slow response in these tests, when studied along with results of MRI, spinal tap and neurological tests, can help diagnose MS. Seventy-seven percent of people with a definite MS diagnosis and 67% of people with probable MS have abnormal SSEP test results.

Finding Your Way

In a healthy body, the signal sent from the brain to the body takes the path that is shortest and surest, so to arrive as quickly as possible. It's as if you were driving home: the route you take is the fastest and safest. When MS is present, your way home has been compromised, just as if you were trying to drive there on a rainy night. The conditions impede your progress, in a way very similar to the demyelization or stripping of nerve endings associated with MS. The signal is trying to find its way from the brain to the body, but your ability to send and receive the messages just doesn't exist.

However, through consistent repetitive exercise, the nerve signal finds a new connection and potentially even other pathways to follow. I believe this is how my clients have achieved their progress. Even though at first it was difficult, as long as they kept trying, they found their way.

Even after MRI, MRS, MTI, DTI, fMRI, and spinal tap are performed, neurologists are reluctant to diagnosis MS if only one episode has occurred, primarily because there are other causes of demyelination that sometimes occur only once. That is why at least two episodes of demyelination separated by at least a month and in two distinct locations in the CNA have to occur for neurologists to consider MS as a possible cause. Several months or even years may pass before a positive diagnosis of MS can be made.

Will the MS will be benign or malignant?

Once MS has been diagnosed, doctors try to determine whether it will be benign or malignant. It's hard to tell with certainty, but there are indicators at the onset of the disease that help doctors predict whether the MS will develop into a benign or malignant form. Generally, sensory symptoms that are present along with motor and/or coordination symptoms at onset foretell a more benign disease course than if motor and/or coordination symptoms appear unaccompanied by sensory symptoms. Most people with MS have a form of the disease that is somewhere between benign and malignant. And past history with the disease seems to be a good indicator of future developments. This means that someone who has had a slowly progressing form of MS will probably continue to have a slowly progressing form.

Benign Disease Course
- Initial symptoms are purely sensory or optic neuritis.
- A long interval between the first two relapses.
- Disease onset before the age of 25.
- Few lesions show on the MRI scan.
- Low number of affected neurological systems five years after onset.

- Low neurological deficit score five years after onset.
- High degree of remission from the last relapse.
- The absence of myelin basic protein (MBP) in the cerebrospinal fluid (CSF) during remissions.
- Onset symptoms from only one as opposed to various regions.
- Female sex.

Malignant Disease Course
- A greater number of neurological areas affected at onset.
- Many lesions showing on MRI scan at onset.
- Pyramidal, cerebellar, and sphincter involvement at onset.
- Coordination symptoms at onset.
- Progressive disease course at onset.
- Oligoclonal banding in spinal tap present in the early phases of the disease.
- Disease onset after 40 years of age.
- Less than one-year interval between the first two relapses.
- Motor symptoms affected at onset.
- Brainstem involvement at onset.
- Male sex.

The Kurtze Expanded Disability Status Scale (EDSS)

The Kurtze Expanded Disability Status Scale is a numerical system devised to measure the severity of the disability one is suffering as a result of MS. Evaluation is based upon symptoms observed during a neurological examination. The observations are classified into eight functional systems (FSs): pyramidal, cerebellar, brainstem, sensory, bowel and bladder, visual, cerebral.

EDDS

Level Description

0.0   Normal neurological function.

1.0   No disability, minimal signs in one functional system (FS).

1.5   No disability, minimal signs in one FS.

2.0   Minimal disability in one FS.

2.5   Mild disability in one FS or minimal disability in two FS.

3.0   Moderate disability in one FS, or mild disability in three or four FS. Fully ambulatory.

3.5   Fully ambulatory but with moderate disability in one FS and more than minimal disability in several others.

4.0   Fully ambulatory without aid, self-sufficient, out of bed for twelve hours a day and able to walk 500 yards without rest or help.

4.5   Fully ambulatory without aid, out of bed most of the day, able to work a full day, requires some assistance, able to walk 300 yards with help.

5.0   Ambulatory without help. Can walk about 200 yards without aid or rest. Disability does impair many daily activities.

5.5   Ambulatory without assistance or rest or help. Disability precludes full daily activities.

6.0   Needs assistance such as canes, crutches, braces in order to walk 100 yards without help or resting.

6.5   Needs constant assistance (canes, crutches, braces) to walk 20 yards without aid.

7.0   Unable to walk 5 yards without aid. Wheelchair is required for most of the day, yet is able to transfer self in and out of wheelchair. Out of bed for 12 hours a day.

7.5   Unable to take more than a few steps. Restricted to wheelchair, which may have to be motorized. Out of bed most of day and performs most bodily functions without aid.

8.0   Mostly restricted to bed or a chair or wheelchair. Still performs many self-care functions, and still has function of arms.

8.5   Restricted to bed most of the day, has some use of arms and performs some self-care activities.

9.0   Confined to bed. Can still communicate and eat.

9.5   Unable to communicate or eat. Confined to bed.

10.0   Death.

Conclusion

Even with all of the modern medical technology available today, you can see that we still do not have a definitive way to determine when or even if a person has contracted MS. As amazing as that may seem, it's no wonder there are so much mystery, fear, and even shame associated with this disease. There are many persons who would rather make up stories to explain their health problems instead of telling the truth about an MS diagnosis.

Most of my MS clients tell stories of having the disease for years before it was actually diagnosed by a physician. They knew something was not the way it was supposed to be, but they lived in fear of what else they might have.

Because it is hard to rely on the medical community to get the whole story of MS, many of my clients were left on their own to find solutions, and that is how I met most of them. They chose not to settle for what their doctors told them to accept (to be happy with the time they had as long as they could and make the most of it while they could still walk). This defeatist attitude certainly wasn't like that of the MS patients I've encountered. All of them were all absolutely determined not to give up but to fight MS with everything possible. This strength of will is what inspired me to search for new answers for them.

It is important for me to state that I do not intend or want to undermine the need for proper medical care. I would not have sought out Dr. Thrower's expertise otherwise. My intention is instead to show the importance of being proactive as opposed to being reactive (as conventional medicine dictates). I realize that there is a shift in the manner in which medical students are being taught to address this issue; however, the delay in achieving real-world results will take years before today's patients see anything.

The MS patients I have as clients are searching for viable solutions now.

Because MS has so many symptoms, it's very hard to diagnose and treat effectively. The disease affects everyone in a different way. It is rarely the same from patient to patient. This is a problem, because this is what science bases factual findings on: through studies where different individuals share similar symptoms, which simply doesn't happen for MS patients.

This is why the approach I took worked: I was able to take each person on, no matter at what stage his or her disease happened to be. We took on one symptom at a time until all their conditions and issues were addressed.

3

Treatment of Multiple Sclerosis

There is no cure for MS, only treatments to slow the progression of the disease and lessen its effects and symptoms. This chapter explores the new drug and treatment options that are being researched and made available today.

Beta Interferon
Beta interferon is a genetically engineered copy of proteins that occur naturally in the human body. They reduce the level of gamma interferon, which is associated with the onset and progression of MS. They also seem to prevent white blood cells from attacking myelin, keep Tcells from releasing cytokines that encourage inflammation, and impede immune system cells from rushing to the inflammation site. Beta interferon can be associated with post-injection flu-like achiness. Worsening of headaches and depression

has also been reported. Blood counts and liver function studies should be monitored periodically while on beta interferon therapy.

Glatiramer Acetate

Glatiramer Acetate is a collection of synthetic peptide string derivatives that prevent T cells from attacking and destroying myelin. Glatiramer acetate is molecularly similar to myelin basic protein. It shifts developing T-cells towards a more protective, regulatory type of cell. These cells have anti-inflammatory and protective effects in the brain itself. Side effects include mild inflammation at the injection site. More serious side effects are flushing, chest and joint pains, weakness, nausea, anxiety, and muscle stiffness. These usually do not last longer than 15 minutes.

Steroids

The prescription of steroids, hormones produced by the human body, is another approach that some neurologists are using to treat people with MS, particularly those displaying predominantly motor rather than sensory symptoms. Glucocorticosteroids, mineralcorticosteroids, androgens, and progestins are all types of steroids, although glucocorticosteroids are most commonly used to treat MS relapses. It should be noted that although steroids such as cortisone are effective in reducing the immediate impact of relapses, they are ineffective in stopping the progression of MS. That's not to mention their significant side effects, which include acne, weight gain, seizures, psychosis, depression, headaches, fatigue, growth of facial hair, nausea, vomiting, and adrenal insufficiency.

Other Immunotherapies

Total lymphoid irradiation: The lymph nodes are irradiated with small doses of X-rays over the course of several weeks. The intent is to destroy lymphoid tissue, which is actively involved in the destruction of tissue in autoimmune diseases such as MS. Trial results for this procedure are inconclusive so far, and side effects are potentially dangerous.

Monoclonal antibodies: Monoclonal antibodies are like designer molecules. They are developed to block key steps in various autoimmune diseases and in some cancers. Natulizumate was approved for use in the USA in June of 2006, although safety concerns persist.

Plasmapheresis (blood plasma exchange): Blood is removed from the patient, and the plasma is separated from the parts of the blood that could contain antibodies and other immunologically active matter. The isolated plasma is then returned to the patient. This procedure remains at the clinical testing stage.

Bone marrow transplantation: Bone marrow is transplanted into patients who have undergone drug or radiation therapy to suppress their immune system. Severe side effects may result.

Intravenous immunoglobulin: Derived from human antibodies, this therapy has been used as both a therapy for acute attacks and as long-term therapy to reduce relapse rates and slow progression of disability.

Antigen Therapy

Scientists searching for an MS vaccine removed myelin-attacking T cells from animals, infected them with experimental allergic encephalomyelitis (EAE), inactivated the T cells, then injected them back into the animals. This resulted in destruction of the immune system cells that were attacking the myelin. In limited trials, scientists have tested a similar vaccine in humans and noticed no side effects.

Peptide Therapy

Peptide therapy is similar to antigen therapy in that it is based upon evidence that the body, if helped, can muster an immune response against the T cells that destroy myelin. To induce a response strong enough to kill the errant T cells, a peptide from the T cell is isolated and injected into the body. The immune system treats this injected peptide as an invader and launches an attack on any myelin-destroying T cells that carry the peptide.

Blocking Cytokines

Scientists are studying substances that may block harmful cytokines, as well as way to produce protective cytokines.

Immune suppressants: Various immune suppressants are used in MS, mainly in more difficult to treat cases. Mitoxantrone is the only FDA-approved option.

Therapy to Improve Nerve Impulse Conduction

Because MS disrupts the transmission of electrochemical messages between the brain and body, researchers are investigating medications to improve the conduction of nerve impulses. It has been noted that demyelinated nerves show abnormal potassium activity. Therefore scientists are studying drugs that block the channels through which potassium moves. By doing this, they hope to restore conduction of nerve impulses.

Remyelination

Some scientists are focusing on ways to reverse the damage to myelin and oligodendrocytes, the cells that manufacture and maintain myelin in the central nervous system. Since scientists already know that oligodendrocytes form new myelin after an attack, they are investigating ways to stimulate this reaction. Studies of animals indicate that monoclonal antibodies and certain immunosuppressant drugs may speed remyelination.

4-Aminopyridine

This investigational drug improves electrical conduction in demyelinated nerve fibers. It may help with heat sensitivity and with exertional weakness. Caution should be used in people at risk for seizures.

Unproven Therapies

Because MS is a disease for which there is no universally effective treatment and no known cause, many unsubstantiated claims of cures have been made over the years. A partial list of these "therapies" includes: injections of snake venom, electrical stimulation of the spinal cord's dorsal column, removal of the thymus gland, breathing pressurized (hyperbaric) oxygen in a special chamber, injections of beef heart and hog pancreas extracts, intravenous or oral calcium orotate (calcium EAP), hysterectomy, removal of dental fillings containing silver or mercury amalgams, bee sting therapy, various "cellular" infusions, and surgical implantation of pig brain into the patient's abdomen. None of these treatments has been found to be effective for MS or any of its symptoms.

New Research

Much recent research has focused on looking for the genes that make some people susceptible to MS. These "genetic markers" are variations in genes that may contribute to the onset and progression of MS. Particular attention is being paid to genetic mutations that may result in a proclivity or predisposition to MS, as well as to the way genes interact with viruses, diet, climate, and other factors. The genetic history of families is also being traced in order to better understand hereditary factors in MS. Particular focus is on genes that govern the immune system.

Since women get MS almost twice as frequently as men, studies are also focusing on chromosome 12, which contains genes that control the powerful immune messenger chemical called gamma interferon (IFN). IFN gamma has been found to be much more active in women with MS than in men with MS.

Ethnicity is another factor that interests MS researchers. One study now under way involves collection of genetic material from a large number of ethnically diverse families of MS patients. The aim of the study is to determine if DNA abnormalities may be responsible for MS in these populations.

Haplotype mapping is yet another approach being explored. Haplotypes are blocks of genes found on chromosomes. Once the "Hapmap" is complete, researchers will be able to use it to compare the haplotype patterns of people with MS to those of people without MS.

In a large ongoing study, MS lesions in brain tissues are being examined to identify the types of immune cells and other immune factors responsible for tissue destruction. The questions the study hopes to answer are: What causes an MS lesion to develop? Why do people with MS differ in the type of lesion they develop? Why is myelin the target of immune attacks in some people with MS while in others the myelin-making cells (oligodendrocytes) are targeted? What is the relationship between the different types of lesions that occur in people with MS and the different ways these groups of people respond to treatment? What is the relationship between the four lesion types and differences seen on MRI scans or in DNA samples?

Conclusion

The work I have done with my MS clients is not a substitute for their proper medical treatments, or even a new alternative theory promising to cure their disease. I have always said to my clients, I am not a doctor and I am not trying to play one.

I have recently heard that some physicians have begun to give training/workout advice as though prescribing a drug treatment. It's important, however, to find a personal trainer who is qualified in this field. Certification does not mean qualification. There are literally hundreds of personnel trainer certification associations in existence today; unfortunately, what does not yet exist is a standardization of care.

Another common complaint from my MS clients is that they don't want to be reliant on drug treatments as a means of living their life and keeping their symptoms at bay. Because of that, and because of the high cost of prescription drugs and side effects of these medications, a lot of people with MS are looking for alternative treatments.

These are only some of the reasons why the MS patients who worked with me were searching for something to work with their treatments and to give them hope. What my program became was a way for them to learn to create something that they never knew existed: a way to take ownership of their health and well-being.

4

Treatment of Symptoms

While some scientists are researching ways to prevent and treat MS itself, others arc looking for new and better medications to control the symptoms of MS. The following are some of the symptoms and treatments for them.

Spasticity

Many people with MS experience muscle spasticity, primarily in their lower limbs. It is usually treated with muscle relaxants and tranquilizers. Baclofen, the most commonly prescribed medication for this symptom, may be taken orally. For more severe cases, a surgically implanted pump can deliver a liquid form of Baclofen directly into the spinal fluid. Tizanidine, used for years in Europe and now approved in the United States, appears to function similarly to baclofen. Diazepam, clonazepam, and dantrolene can also reduce spasticity. Physical therapy is also useful, and it can help prevent irreversible contractures, or shortening of muscles. Therapists may give instructions for home stretching exercises, one way to decrease symptoms from spasticity. Injections of botulinum toxin may reduce spasticity in selected muscles. Surgery to reduce spasticity is rarely used in MS.

Author Tip

I used to address spasticity with a work/rest/work technique with resistance training, making sure to take a proper rest break after each and every set of an exercise for the working muscle group. Sometimes it was also necessary to rest or pause right in the middle of performing a set in order to be able to finish the exercise.

Weakness and Ataxia (incoordination)

Weakness and incoordination are also common in people with MS. Spasticity can actually be beneficial in cases of weakness, as it lends support to weak limbs by increasing muscle tone. In such cases, medications that alleviate spasticity completely may be inappropriate. Physical therapy and exercise can also help preserve remaining function, as well as various aids such as foot braces, canes, and walkers. Physicians can occasionally provide temporary relief from weakness, spasms, and pain by injecting a drug called phenol into the spinal cord, muscles, or nerves in the arms or legs.

Optic neuritis

Optic neuritis (a relapse involving visual pathways) is common in MS. Symptoms usually improve with time, although infusions of intravenous steroids, methylprednisolone, may speed recovery. Visual symptoms can also include double vision (diplopia) or bouncy eye movements (nystagmus).

Fatigue

Fatigue is among the most common of MS symptoms. There are many types and causes of fatigue. Lassitude is a sense of sudden, overwhelming tiredness. Nerve fiber fatigue is weakness brought on with exertion or excessive heat. It is important to know that symptoms brought on by heat or exercise are not an indication of new damage and are only temporary. Energy levels are also affected by your mood, overall health, and medications. Exercise has been shown to decrease fatigue. Medication options for lassitude management include amantidine, modafinil, and stimulants (like those used for ADHD). As mentioned earlier, 4-aminopyridine may help with nerve fiber fatigue. Some antidepressants may boost energy levels while also dealing with any component of depression.

Pain

Pain is more common than previously appreciated in MS. Pain can manifest as burning, tingling, facial pains (trigeminal neuralgia), or painful spasms. Physical therapy may help with some aches and pains, especially those associated with increased muscle tone or back/neck pain. Medications for pain include anti-inflammatory drugs like ibuprofen, anti-depressants, anti-convulsants, and sometimes opiate analgesics. Severe pain may require more aggressive measures like pain pumps to deliver drugs into the spinal fluid or spinal cord stimulators.

Bladder malfunctions

Bladder problems often develop as MS progresses. In some people, the bladder is small and wants to empty all the time, while in others, the bladder is large and empties poorly. Sometimes the valve or sphincter of the bladder doesn't seem to want to open and let urine out. Symptoms include urinary frequency, urgency, incontinence, and urinary tract infections. Treatment focuses on avoiding bladder irritants like caffeine and aspartame. Ironically, some people actually worsen their bladder symptoms by restricting fluid intake. Concentrated urine can act as a bladder irritant as well. There are many medications that help with a small, overactive bladder, fewer for urinary retention. Retention may require catheterization to empty the bladder. Bladder infections require antibiotics. A newer surgically implanted "pacemaker" for the bladder, may be an option for treating the large, poorly emptying bladder.

Constipation

Constipation is frequently a result of MS patients' not drinking enough fluids because of urinary problems they are experiencing. Drinking more water and adding fiber to the diet usually alleviates this condition. Bowel function usually improves with exercise.

Sexual Dysfunction

Sexual dysfunction can result from MS, especially in patients with urinary problems. Men may experience occasional erection failure. Penile implants, injection of papaverine, and electrostimulation are methods used to remedy the problem. Women may experience insufficient lubrication or have difficulty reaching orgasm. Oral medications, penile implants, vaginal gels, and vibrating devices may be helpful in these cases. Counseling, especially in the absence of urinary problems, is also helpful, particularly since psychological factors can also cause these symptoms. Depression, for instance, can intensify symptoms of fatigue, pain, and sexual dysfunction. In these cases, antidepressants and anti-anxiety medications may be prescribed.

Tremors

Although often resistant to physical therapy, tremors can sometimes be treated with drugs. Surgery is used in extreme cases.

Drugs Used to Treat Symptoms of Multiple Sclerosis

Symptom	Drug
Spasticity	Baclofen (Lioresal)
	Tizanidine (Zanaflex)
	Diazepam (Valium)
	Clonazepam (Klonopin)
	Dantrolene (Dantrium)

Symptom	Drug
Optic neuritis	Methylprednisolone (Solu-Medrol)
	Oral steroids
Fatigue	Antidepressants
	Amantadine (Symmetrel)
	Modafinil (Provigil)
	Methylphenidate (Ritalin)
Pain	Anti-inflammatory drugs (aspirin, acetaminophen, ibuprofen)
	Antidepressants
	Opiate analgesics
	Anti-convulsants
Trigeminal neuralgia	Carbamazapine, other anticonvulsants
Sexual dysfunction	Papaverine injections (in men)
	Oral medications (Viagra, Levitra, Cialis)

Physical Fatigue

Physical fatigue is the most common aspect of MS that my clients experience. At one time or another, they have all told me that their fatigue lowered their quality of life the most.

Physical fatigue is simply a constant energy expenditure on the body, 24/7. Because of this, any additional energy demanded over and above the average daily use will naturally take a larger toll on an MS patient. Thus it is absolutely imperative that you not waste any energy, because there is not a lot to spare. Train smarter, not harder. Those with MS must work out in a manner that makes the most of their limited extra energy. The goal is to learn to train at maximum efficiency, and to receive more and do less. This is possible only through workouts that are safe and effective. As an added bonus, these are also safer!

Another complicated issue is MS patients' heat sensitivity. For a long time those with MS were instructed to avoid physical exercise because it would lead to overheating. This broad statement discouraged a lot of people from participating in physical activity, even though we know that it is good for your overall health and well-being.

There is an assumption that for exercising to have any beneficial effect on the body, you must break a sweat or be short of breath. This isn't true, as many recent studies have documented the positive effects of low-to-moderate exercise. These studies were done for everyone, not just MS patients!

Once again, this leads us back to learning how to train at maximum efficiency, or gaining more by doing less. Not only is this possible; if you have MS, it is imperative.

There have been occasions in training when clients began to overheat, but we handled this by setting a very specific tempo in our workouts. Whenever this happened, we stopped momentarily to allow the body's core temperature to lower. If this did not work fast enough, we would place a cold wet towel on the forehead or the back of their neck. The changing seasons also affected this heightened sensitivity, so it is important to be indoors in an air-conditioned environment. The training facility I used had a great cooling system, so it was always cold, and my clients loved it.

Setting the tempo was also used to establish rest periods after every set of every exercise during the entire workout session. How my client felt that day—whether it was a bad or good day—would determine the length of the rest (anywhere from 45 seconds to 1½ minutes). This ensured they would have enough stamina to make it to the end of the workout.

This kind of training did wonders on improving my clients' general conditioning levels, as well as establishing a baseline fitness level. Soon they were achieving predetermined short-, mid-, and long-term physical goals. This development of higher stamina levels is key to achieving success and what this book is all about.

Conclusion

The various symptoms of MS have always posed endless challenges to my clients, to say the least, but as long as they remained determined and kept a positive attitude, almost anything was possible. (This attitude and determination are essential to achieving realistic results, and you will find this mental approach outlined later in Chapter 9.)

One of the most common issues with spasticity is that it eventually simply stops MS patients from moving completely: Their muscles would seize up for no reason. A single muscle contraction takes a tremendous amount of coordination that most people do not realize until the moment their muscles do not respond to their simplest physical demands.

It's essential to regularly require your muscles to contract, relax, and contract again. In other words: performing consistent resistance training workouts. I don't refer to this in the traditional sense of weight lifting to gain strength. However, resistance placed upon the body using body weight, free weights, dumbbells, body bars, machines, or whatever you may have on hand, requires the muscles to perform. I always say, "A little is a lot" to my clients, who have wondered on occasion if the small amount of work they were doing was doing any good. Yet, after the workout, they would tell me their muscles felt a little tired and fatigued—but not sore. "Like you had used them?" Yes, they answered. That's exactly what you want to happen. Exercise does not have to hurt in order for it to give you its benefits.

What I found most interesting were the results of the clients who came to me with spasticity as their main problem. After beginning consistent resistance training, they reported either that spasticity ceased to occur or that when it did occur, it was not as bad as previous incidents. While I cannot make claims that resistance training stops spasticity, I will say that as far as my clients are concerned, there was a dramatic and very real impact. How was this possible? How did they increase physical strength and decrease spasticity and weakness, while suffering from MS? The simple answer is that their hard work paid off.

I often say, "If you work—it works." Having MS did not keep my clients from taking an active role in their care or from fighting against MS. All of my clients knew why and how they were going to work out and exactly what they would be required to accomplish before they began. This, while time-consuming at first, does pay off in the end. It's like the old adage: "If you're going to try and do something—do it right or don't do it at all."

5

The Benefits
of Exercise

It is well known that regular exercise and increased physical activity can both add years to your life and improve the quality of those years. In general, the more exercise you do, the greater the benefits will be. Cardiorespiratory endurance, muscle strength, muscle endurance, flexibility, and body composition are all improved by various exercises.

Long-Term Benefits of Exercise

- Decreased risk of heart disease. Inactive people are twice as likely to develop coronary artery disease (CAD) as active people.
- Decreased blood pressure. High blood pressure increases the risk of heart disease, stroke, and kidney disease. Inactive people are twice as likely to develop high blood pressure as active people.
- Decreased body fat. Regular physical activity helps maintain optimal body weight and composition. High blood pressure increases the risk of heart disease, stroke, and kidney disease.

- Decreased cholesterol level. A high blood cholesterol level increases the risk of heart disease. Regular exercise raises the level of "good" cholesterol and lowers the level of "bad" cholesterol.
- Decreased risk of diabetes. Physical activity lowers the risk of type 2 diabetes and increases glucose uptake for those who already have diabetes.
- Decreased risk of cancer. Physical activity lowers the risk of colon and breast cancer.
- Decreased risk of osteoporosis. Regular exercise delays bone loss and promotes bone formation.
- Decreased arthritis symptoms. Regular exercise helps keep joints flexible and helps build muscle to support the joint.
- Decreased number of sick days. Exercisers feel sick almost 30 percent less often than nonexercisers.
- Decreased chance of premature death. Fit people live longer than unfit people.

Short-Term Benefits

- Physical activity reduces mental and muscular tension and, at the same time, increases concentration and energy level.
- Physical activity provides a break from the daily routine. It's like a minivacation—you're allowed to have fun.
- Physical activity increases self-esteem and self-confidence.
- Though many people start a physical activity program for its long-term benefits, it's the short-term benefits that keep them motivated to continue the habit.

Although exercise for people with MS is more difficult than it is for people without MS, and also potentially more dangerous, few if any doctors dispute its value for countering the fatigue, weakness, and lack of coordination that plagues most patients to some degree.

Additionally, and perhaps most important, exercise helps to combat depression, which many people with MS suffer from.

A 1996 study done at the University of Utah by Jack Petajan, MD, PhD, found that regular aerobic exercise, vigorous enough to raise the pulse and respiration rate, increased fitness, muscle strength, and workout capacity and improved bowel and bladder control in people with multiple sclerosis. Participants in the study also reported reduced depression, fatigue, anxiety, and anger. Other studies have shown that exercise eases spasticity and poor balance in people with MS while increasing cardiovascular capacity.

Exercise is important and necessary no matter what level of MS a person has. Resistive, aerobic, and stretching, are the three main types of exercises beneficial to MS patients. Resistive training makes use of weights, springs, and bands. They increase muscle power and ability and help large muscles burn fat. Resistive exercises can be divided into two categories: isotonic and isometric. In isotonic exercises, the muscles exert force while moving. Isometric exercises involve a muscle that is stationary while exerting force. Resistive exercises should be done carefully, and isometric exercises can tighten muscles, especially spastic ones, too much.

Aerobic exercises work the heart and lungs and increase stamina. Stair climbing, walking, jogging, dancing, swimming, and bicycling are all examples of aerobic activities. MS patients are recommended not to push too hard, though. Overexertion can cause exhaustion, injuries and sleep disruption. Morning is the best time of day to exercise for this reason. In fact, it has been found that morning exercise routines improve sleep patterns in people with MS.

Stretching is especially helpful for muscles that will be exercised, and it helps prevent injuries caused by sudden muscle elongation. It also fights the spasticity, increases the range of motion in joints, and prevents muscle contracture.

Rest periods between exercise routines are critical, as is a slow start. Exercise intensity should increase gradually, but your limits should not be exceeded. Thirty to sixty minutes a day, four times a week, is ideal.

No discussion about exercise would be complete without discussion of diet, which provides the fuel for exercise. There seems to be a general consensus amongst researchers that a low-fat diet is beneficial if you have MS. Diets low in saturated fats, sucrose, and gluten, and high in linoleic acid, antioxidants, plant protein such as soy, vitamins B12, C, and E, flaxseed oil, and fish have all been touted over the years.

One study supporting this involved 144 multiple sclerosis patients who ate a low-fat diet for 34 years. For each of three categories of neurological disability (minimum, moderate, severe), patients who stuck to the prescribed diet (less than or equal to 20 grams of fat per day) demonstrated significantly less deterioration and much lower death rates than did those who consumed more fat than prescribed (greater than 20 grams of fat per day). The greatest benefit was seen in those with minimum disability at the start of the trial; in this group, when those who died from non-MS diseases were excluded from the analysis, 95 percent survived and remained physically active.

Conclusion

As you've just read, the effects that various types of exercises have to improve the ability to combat MS and the overall quality of life is well documented. However, I have come to the conclusion, based on my interactions with many MS groups, that most MS patients do not work out. Either they are afraid of hurting themselves, or their doctors do not encourage them to try to work out.

This is why Dr. Thrower and I saw eye to eye from the first time we met. We agreed that MS patients need to find some kind of physical exercise that appeals to them, as well as seek out a qualified fitness professional to help them work out and keep them motivated.

There are many misconceptions that surround exercise for MS patients. There is no single standard of care. If you are looking for a physical trainer, please consider seeking a professional who also carries the title of PRS (postrehabilitation specialist).

Postrehabiliation training is specifically tailored to the individual, taking into account MS symptoms and to what stage the person's disease has progressed. The very nature of MS is that it's different for each patient, so this individualized care gives them the kind of attention and care they deserve. Postrehab is about going beyond where you are now to where you want to be in the future.

These three D's—Drive, Desire, and Determination—are the central motivating ideals my clients possessed. The direction I provided was not only the workout sessions, but also physical education. Knowing the ways the body operates and its functions allows for compensation for a disorder such as MS.

When one aspect of the body has been compromised, the opposing muscles and joints have to bear the extra burden. The most common physical injury is one that occurs over time. You could be unaware of the damage you are doing each time you perform an exercise incorrectly, until it is too late. Usually this means undergoing a surgical procedure to solve the situation.

With MS clients, the largest thing I noticed was their overcompensation while walking. They had a wobbly gait, and this told me everything I need to know. (For instance, if they had a dropped foot on the left side, their right side knee and hip would bear the majority of the body's weight. Over time, this would lead to an overuse injury to their right leg or right hip, and would create the possibility of total loss of mobility.) That is why a total-body training approach is so important. A PRS will see the connection between the left and right sides of the body, as well as the client's entire physical well-being. In Postrehab, we can address the real issues of our clients in creating an exercise program that is safe and effective and that they can follow for the rest of their lives.

Part II: Exercises for Multiple Sclerosis

6

Gait Analysis

Most of the MS clients I have worked with had problems walking correctly. They experienced partial loss of mobility in the lower extremities and difficulty maintaining a straight course, and I would observe them literally stumbling, limping, and moving from one place to the other by any means possible.

This was not completely their fault, as much of the MS literature says to avoid any risk of wearing yourself out (i.e., the fatigue factor). It also suggests whenever possible to take elevators or escalators or use power chairs. I realize this advice is intended to help, but by failing to physically challenge yourself on a regular basis, your body will deteriorate, potentially resulting in a complete loss of mobility.

It All Started by Taking a Walk

My sessions with MS clients would begin with reteaching them how to walk correctly, literally one step at a time. I would first observe them walking naturally, six to eight steps at a time, which would allow me to see how their body weight was transferred and thus what their issues might be. Once I was able to identify their main walking error (from a dropped foot, weakened leg, typically below the knee, or even a problem with their vision), they could relearn how to walk. They would repeat those same six to eight steps, back and forth, over and over again, until new patterns of movement began to emerge.

The intention of this aspect of the exercise was to apply the new walking technique by creating improved motor pathways. As I mentioned earlier, the only way the human body learns is through repetitive motion, and how you repeat an action becomes how it will be recalled in the future and how it is programmed into the muscle memory.

At the core of this technique is concentrating on how the heels of the feet would come in contact with the floor. It's crucial that the heel of the foot make contact with the floor on the very first step, as it sets up the entire movement of the walking stride. Many MS patients step and make the first connection with their toes (classic dropped foot), which doesn't provide enough stability. As soon as my clients began walking heel first, they would report to me that their incidents of falling dramatically decreased or even stopped altogether. This is a perfect example of why a movement done effectively is also safer.

The next part of the foot movement is rolling through the foot onto the ball, then onto the toes, which are responsible for propelling the body forward. The ball of the foot is a main joint involved in the mechanics of the walk, but is not given much attention. However, let me stress the effect this can have on your walking technique; it proved invaluable to my clients. The toes not only provide the propelling power but allow you to feel secure with the surface because of the toes' sensitivity. I connected this to some of my clients' habit of walking around barefoot when at home. However, it is a good idea to use supportive shoes the rest of the time.

The last instruction I give is to slow down. A lot is going on during every step, and walking correctly requires time and concentration. Try to slow your pace down as you relearn how to walk all over again.

Some of the other mistakes I noticed when observing my clients included:

- Drifting off to one side during the walking exercise (usually compensating for MS by overuse of unaffected areas). This is a classic overcompensating walk that can lead to other orthopedic issues.
- A duck walk, with the feet deliberately turned out to provide greater security. I had a client who told me that her doctor had instructed her to walk this way so that she would feel more secure while walking. I do not agree with this.

Walking Exercises

The best way to maintain proper biomechanics and walk safely and effectively is to maintain a straight posture. You should have your hips directly over your thighs, and this straight posture should continue down through the kneecap, the shin/ankle, and between your third and fourth toes (numbering your pinky toe as the first toe). This way the weight of your body is carried by the strongest points possible: the center of the joints. This allows the larger muscles of the hips and quads to do their jobs.

You should also be conscious of your core. By contracting your abs while walking, you are connecting the upper body to the lower body. You should also always keep your head up and look in the direction you are moving. It's a common practice of many MS patients to look down at the floor for added security, and while I understand the reasons behind this kind of thinking, the surface of the ground is not moving. You are—so concentrate on your body.

To quickly summarize: When you contact the floor, the order should be from heel to ball to toe. Move slowly in a straight path, not drifting from side to side. Tighten your abs and keep your head up.

After practicing these kinds of walking techniques for a considerable period of time, almost every single client reported a dramatic decrease in their falls, trips, and accidents associated with walking. Improved stability and stamina were pleasant side effects, and they achieved a new greater sense of coordination and mobility, which they had not expected to ever get back after being diagnosed as having MS.

Here are a few exercises that may help you when learning to walk again.

Railroad Tracks

Figure Eights

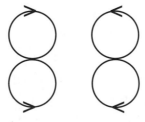

Racetracks

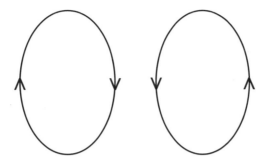

Here are a few illustrations of improper walking.

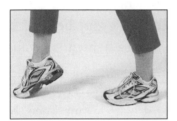
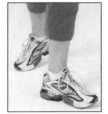
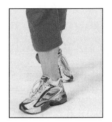

Pictured is the correct way to walk.

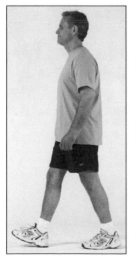
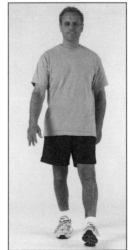

It's a very important part of my philosophy to remain as capable as possible for as long as possible. Here are a few exercises designed to help you with these situations:

Functional Lowering/Standing Technique

It can be a difficult task to get down onto the floor. Stand with your legs apart, one in front of the other (2 to 3 feet apart depending on your stride length). Now begin to lower your body down between both of your legs by bending your knees at right angles. You should be evenly distributing the weight to the front as well as to the back leg. Brace your upper body by placing your hands (arms extended straight) on the front thigh for support. Keep your head up and your spine straight at all times and be sure to tighten your abs to help with stabilization. Lower yourself slowly and in a controlled manner. Do not just drop down on your knees, as this may result in an injury. Once in place, you should be down on one knee. Now place one hand at your side and sit on the floor.

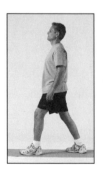 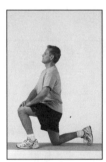 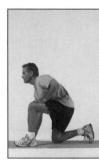 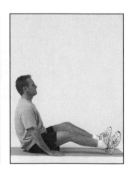

Standing Technique

From a position lying on the ground, roll over onto the left side of your body, and then onto your stomach. Push back with both of your arms until you are resting on your knees. Now bring one leg up so your upper thigh is parallel to the floor while simultaneously bringing your back leg underneath your body at a 90-degree angle to the upper torso. Place your hands on your front thigh and use them to push off to support your weight. Now rise up, keeping your head and spine straight. Make sure to push off from the ball of your back foot to properly propel you to the standing position.

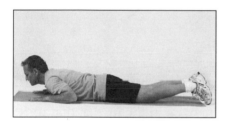
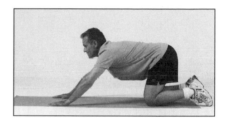

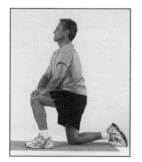
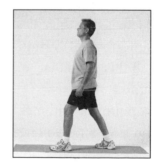

7

Core/Ab Training

It is a mystery to me, even with all the hype in the media, that most people do not yet know how to effectively train their midsection. The problem is that there has not been a consistent message, and in fact, misinformation is running rampant. Many individuals try to sell "the ab this or ab that" on an infomercial, based on unsubstantiated claims.

The amount of gimmicky ab-training products sold each year makes me stop and wonder: What's really going on here? Is the media deliberately taking advantage of the limited knowledge readily available? Remember, you can fool some people some of the time—but you can't fool all of the people all the time. People can tell that they are being sold and as a result have become very skeptical of much of the information out there. In other words, people don't know what or who to believe, so have chosen not to believe in anything at all. This is part of why it's so easy to get frustrated by lack of results.

It's time to end this through real physical education. By learning the truth about your body's natural abilities, you will be empowered to create an exercise routine that is yours alone. It's my responsibility as a properly trained fitness professional to provide accurate information and dispel the misconceptions about core training.

Whenever possible, abdominal exercises should be performed by yourself without an object or machine to help. It's important not to allow an object or device to dictate the exercise's form. Once you know how abdominal muscles contract, you will create an effective core routine that no machine could ever duplicate. There is no need to wonder if it is working, as your abs will tell you how much they are doing.

There were times when my clients could not maintain a particular position to perform the exercise. Because of this, I developed the partner-, bench-, or stability ball–assisted methods. By maintaining just the minimum of pressure and allowing my clients to do as much of the work as possible, they showed an increased capacity to maintain the positions by themselves.

Basic Crunch

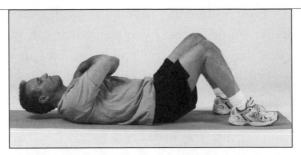

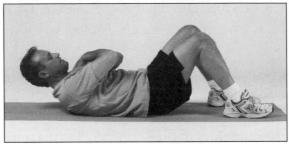

Lie on your back with your knees bent and your feet flat on the floor. Cross your arms across your chest. Do not interlock your hands behind the head as this could lead to a neck injury. Begin by slightly raising your shoulder blades up off the floor. The head and neck should closely follow. Slide the rib cage down toward the pelvis, shortening the distance between them. Do not lift your torso up too high, or rest your shoulder blades onto the floor, until the set is finished.

Advanced Crunch

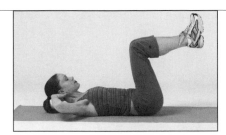 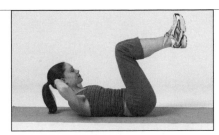

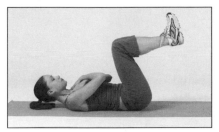 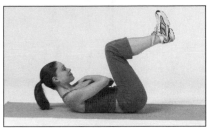

Lie on your back with your knees bent and your feet off the ground, so that your shins form a 90-degree angle with your thighs. Place your hands at your ears and lift your head off the ground. This is the starting position. Slide your chest toward your knees while keeping your feet off the ground and your legs level. Do not cross your ankles, as doing so can pull your lower back. For an easier variation, try crossing your arms across your chest.

Reverse Crunch

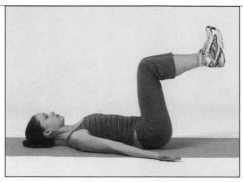

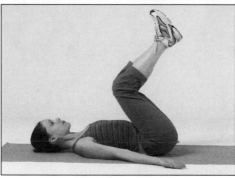

Lie on your back with your knees bent and your feet off the ground, so that your shins form a 90-degree angle with your thighs. Place your arms flat at your sides with your palms up (this discourages you from using your arms for leverage). Raise your pelvis and lower again. Think about rolling your hips toward your sternum, not up toward the sky. You want to keep the movement on a horizontal plane. This exercise will feel as if it is working the lower abs, but it's not excluding the other abdominal areas.

Assisted Advanced Crunch

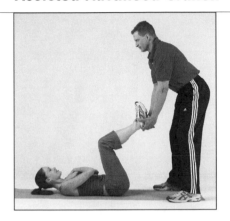 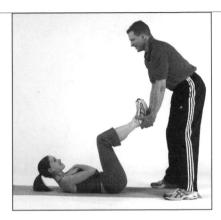

Lie down on your back and place your arms across your chest. Bring your legs up off the floor so that your shins form a 90-degree angle with your thighs. Your partner is holding up the weight of the lower body by cupping the heels in his or her hands. Start your movement by bringing your shoulder blades up off the ground. The head and neck will follow. Perform the crunch motion by shortening the distance between the sternum and the pelvis. Do not lift your waist up towards the ceiling; instead, slide your rib cage down toward your partner. Make sure you do not allow your shoulder blades to make contact with the floor until you have completed the exercise.

Assisted Reverse Crunch

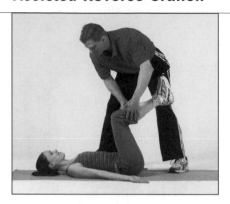 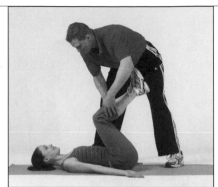

Lie down on your back and place your arms along your sides with the palms facing up. Bring your legs off the floor so that your shins form a 90-degree angle with your thighs. Your partner is holding your legs up by lightly gripping behind the knee joint for support. He will also aid in your rocking/rolling motion of the pelvis back toward your sternum. Make sure that your hips remain flat on the floor. Your partner's assistance should be as minimal as possible.

Advanced Crunch with Bench

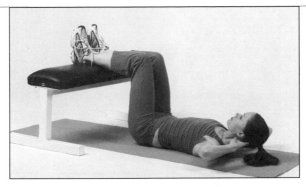

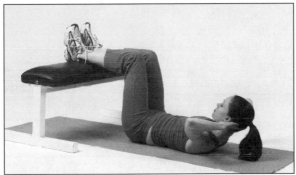

Lie down on your back and place your hands behind your head. Do not interlock your grip; instead, rest the weight of your head on your fingertips. Now lift your legs up so that your ankles are resting on the bench, with a 90-degree angle at your knee joint. Your lower body should remain stationary the entire exercise. Raise your head, neck, and shoulders off the floor slightly. Now slide your rib cage down toward the bench (not up to the ceiling). Once again, make sure you do not allow your shoulder blades to make contact with the floor until you are finished with the set.

Stability Ball Crunch

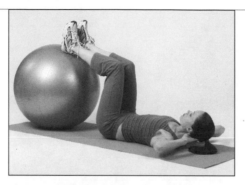

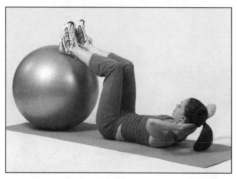

Lie down on your back and place your hands behind your head. Do not interlock your grip; instead, rest the weight of your head on your fingertips. Now lift your legs up so that your ankles are resting on top of the ball, with a 90-degree angle at your knee joint. Be aware that the ball has a tendency to move freely, so extra effort will be needed to control it while performing your crunches. Raise your head, neck, and shoulder blades up off the floor just slightly to establish tension. Now, slide you rib cage down toward the ball (not up to the ceiling). Be careful to keep your shoulder blades off the floor for the entire exercise.

Seated Abdominal Isolation

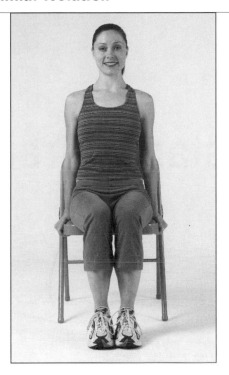

Sit in a chair and relax the upper torso completely, but do not slouch. You will be contracting the abdominals against themselves. This is known as isometric tension. Squeeze the abdominal wall as hard as possible. Be sure not to hold your breath.

8

Resistance Training

In this section I demonstrate a large variety of exercises using free weights, machines, ankle weights, and your own body weight. All of these provide resistance training. This chapter is divided into sections based on the body part being worked.

Lower Body

The following exercises are for beginners and are to be performed after your abdominal workout while still on the mat to help segue into the remainder of the lower body workout.

Single Leg Raise (Quadriceps)

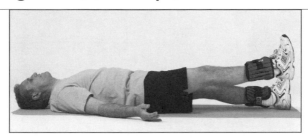

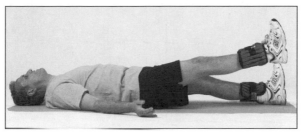

This may be performed with or without ankle weights. Lie on your back with both of your legs extended straight out. Flex your feet so your toes point up towards the ceiling. Place your arms along the side of your body with your palms up. Begin the exercise by raising your right leg up off the floor about 6 to 8 inches (roughly to where your opposite foot's toes are). Hold this position for 10 seconds, and then lower the leg back down to the floor. Switch legs and repeat until you have performed three sets per leg.

To make sure that it's your quadriceps that is doing the work of lifting the leg, always keep your knee slightly flexed or bent. Don't lock your knee joint at any point. To strengthen the abductors or inner thighs, turn your toes so that they point toward the side.

Seated Leg Extension Machine (Quadriceps)

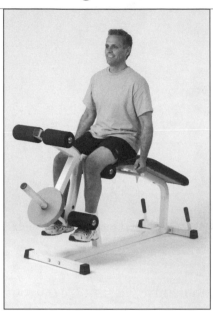 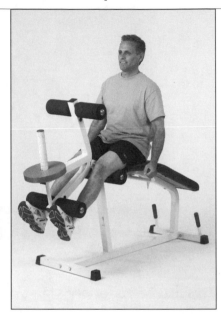

Note: While this is a common piece of gym equipment, it is also often misused. To make sure you are using it properly, sit down at the machine and look down toward the outside of the right knee. You should see an axis pin on the leg extension machine itself. Now imagine a straight line extends out of the axis pin going through the knee joint. This line should pass just behind the rear of the kneecap. The lower shin pad, where you place your legs during exercise, should be just above the ankle joint once your feet are in the flexed position.

You should extend out from your knee joint, not lift upward with the thighs. Grip the seat or handholds with both hands and lift smoothly. Hold the position for 3 to 4 seconds and then lower the weight carefully.

Seated Chair Leg Extension (Quadriceps)

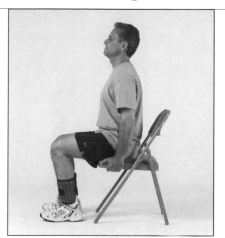 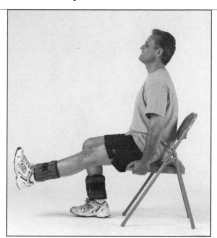

You may perform these with adjustable ankle weights (5 to 10 pounds). Sit on the front half of a stable chair, not on the edge or reclined all the way back. Begin with your knee at a 90-degree angle and your feet flat on the floor. Flex one foot, and then lift it off the floor until it is extended out away from the chair. The angle your leg should make is about 120 degrees. You should never reach 180 degrees of full extension. Make sure that your upper thigh does not lift off of the chair during the extension to keep the pressure on the quads. Take extra care not to lock your knee joint while extending your leg; this is improper form and can lead to injury over time. Try alternating legs at first, and as you progress, attempt extending both simultaneously to increase the intensity of this workout.

Athletic Squat (Quadriceps)

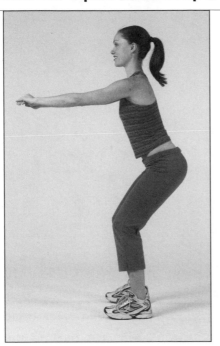 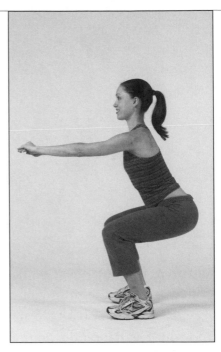

Stand with your feet slightly wider than hip width apart, with your toes pointing straight forward. Clasp your hands and extend your arms out to the front at shoulder-height. Keep your head up and your back straight. Do not bend at the waist or lean forward. Now lower yourself from the hips in a slow and controlled manner, making sure your knees do not extend forward past the toes. Stop when approximately at a 90-degree angle in the knee joint. Try imagining you are sitting back into a chair. Return to an upright position by extending from the hip joint first and the knees last. Do not lock your knees at the top of the movement.

Ballet Squat (Quadriceps)

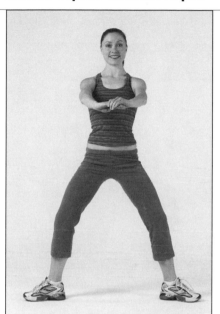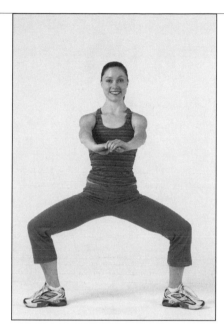

Stand with your feet wider than hip width apart, and your toes pointed out to the sides. Clasp your hands out to the front at shoulder height, tucking your hips under and forward. Your upper body must remain straight and upright for the entire exercise. Now lower yourself down in a slow and controlled manner. Your knees should point out to the sides. Stop when you arrive at a right angle in the knee joint. Now, extend up completely, but do not lock your knees.

One-Legged Squat (Quadriceps)

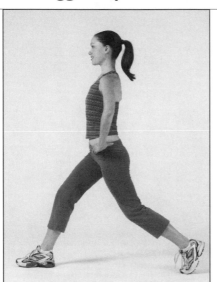 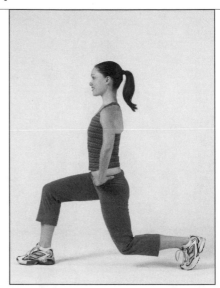

Start with your legs in a staggered stance, one foot in front of the other. Your weight should be evenly distributed between both legs. Now raise yourself up onto the ball of the foot of your back leg and place your hands on your hips. Make sure to keep your upper torso completely still for the entire exercise. Now lower yourself straight down toward the floor so that your weight is evenly distributed between your front and back legs. Be careful with this; don't lunge forward and place more weight on one leg than the other. Stop when your knees create a right angle. Hold the position, then return to the starting position by extending up from your hips. Do not lock your knees.

Quad Stretch (Quadriceps)

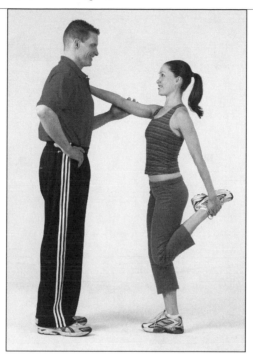

Grab on to a stationary object with one hand and grab your opposite ankle with the other hand. Pull your foot up slightly, keeping your thighs parallel to each other. Hold for 15 seconds and switch sides.

Lying Leg Curls (Hamstrings)

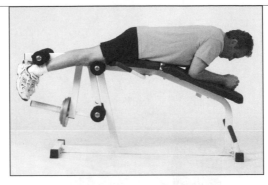

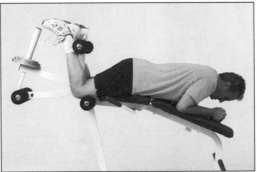

Be sure to position your body with the thigh pad an inch above the kneecap, not resting directly on it. Place your feet under the heel pad with your toes flexed. To stabilize your upper body, contract your abdominals. Don't rest your entire torso on the bench, but instead brace yourself up on your forearms to hold your head and spine straight. Curl your lower leg up toward your glutes, bending your knee joint at a right angle. Now lower the weight until your leg is parallel to the floor. Do not return your leg to a locked position.

Seated Leg Curl Machine (Hamstrings)

If you have the option, use a seated leg curl machine instead of a lying leg curl machine as it is easiest to use with correct form.
Sit down at the machine. Most machines have an adjustable thigh pad that lowers down onto your mid- to upper thigh. Be careful not to let it rest directly on your kneecap. Keep your abdominals contracted for the entire exercise. This will ensure that your lower back is supported and the hips are not engaged. Now curl your leg and end the movement at a 90-degree angle in your knee. When your knee is completely flexed, hold the contraction for one second and squeeze your glutes.

Partner-Assisted Prone Leg Curl (Hamstrings)

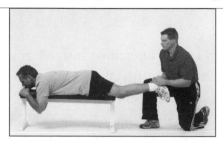 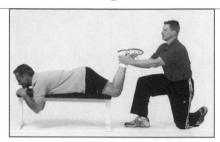

This exercise is more advanced and should be administered only by a trained fitness professional. You can perform this by yourself with no assistance and use ankle weights for resistance.

Lie face down on the floor (or alternatively, on the bench) with your arms resting next to the head (or lightly gripping the sides of the bench). Flex both of your feet as if you were pointing the toes straight down to the floor. Contract your abs and hold them tight during the entire set. Begin by raising both of your feet off of the floor or bench by about 6 inches. Your partner will be cupping the backs of your heels with both hands. Now, lift your lower leg up, bending at the knee as if you were trying to kick yourself in the glutes. Do not exceed a 90-degree angle at your knee joint. Remember, the amount of manual pressure applied by your partner should be slight; you should be aware that he or she is there but not much else. If you sense any pain or tightness in your lower back, stop immediately.

Lying Leg Curl (Hamstrings)

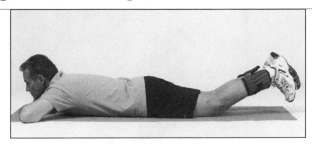

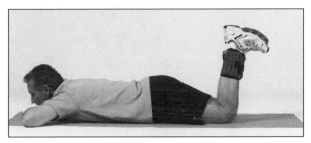

Lie facedown on an exercise mat with your arms along your head. Place your feet together, flexed at the ankles, so that your toes are pointing down into the floor. Begin the movement by bending your knee, bringing your lower leg up toward the glutes. Raise your feet to a 90-degree angle at your knee joint, keeping your upper thigh on the floor. Now squeeze your glutes before lowering your leg back down.

Hamstring Stretch (Hamstrings)

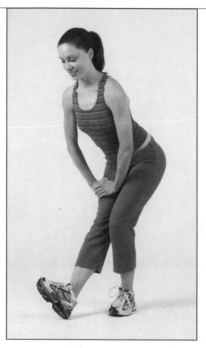

Bend one leg and position the other leg out in front of you as shown. Lean back. Keep the free hand on your thigh. Keep your chest high and your torso upright. Repeat on the opposite side.

Standing Calf Raises (Calves)

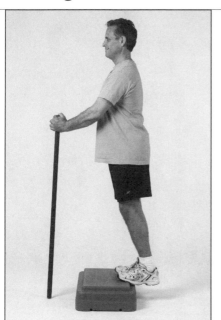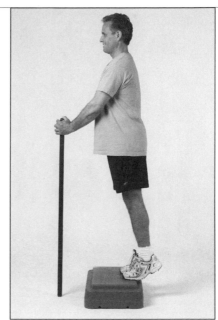

Stand on a raised platform or step. Place your feet about six inches apart, and make sure you are resting on the balls of your feet, not on your toes or instep. Now raise straight up, lifting your heels as high as possible. Pause at the top, then lower yourself back down slowly until you feel a slight stretch in your calves. Make sure not to hold the position excessively at the bottom.

One-Legged Calf Raise (Calves)

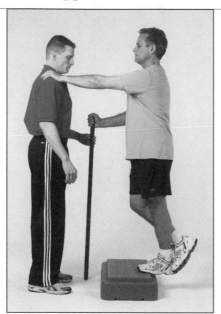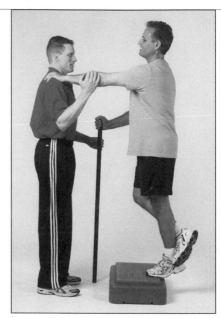

Stand on a raised platform with a partner to help you stay steady. Tuck one foot behind the other's ankle. Now rise up on the ball of the foot as high as possible. Make sure to keep your weight centered. You should stretch only until you feel slight tension in your calf muscle. Lower yourself back down in a controlled manner. Never drop too quickly.

Seated Calf Raise (Calves)

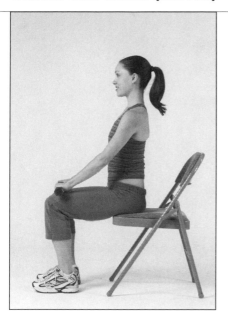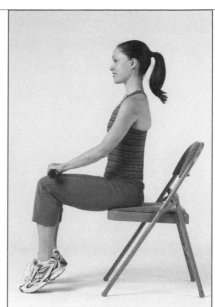

Sit on the side of a bench or the edge of a chair. Place your legs at a right angle with your feet about six inches apart. Rest a pair of dumbbells directly on your thighs near your knee (but not directly on it). Now, rise up onto the balls of your feet. Hold the position, then lower carefully.

Calf Wall Stretch (Calves)

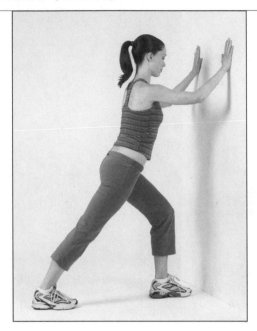

Stand an arm's length away from a wall. Place your hands on the wall, then step forward with one leg, keeping that leg bent. Straighten out your back leg. Keep both of your feet flat on the floor. Now lean forward over the front leg to extenuate the stretch.

Heel Rolls (Anterior Tibialis)

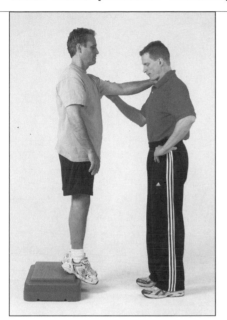 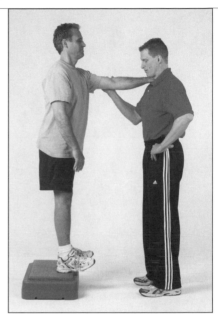

With a partner to help support you, stand with your heels on a block or a raised platform. Let the toes of both of your feet drop down below ankle level. Then pull the toes back up toward your shins as high as possible. Make sure to roll the weight of your body over the center of your ankle joint, using the heel as the fulcrum for this exercise.

Ankle Circles (Ankles)

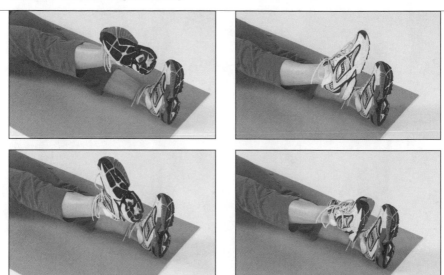

Lie on your back. Turn your toes and ankles to the right, making circular movements. These should begin small at first, then increase to the largest circles possible by the end of the exercise. Now repeat, turning to the left side.

Hip Extension (Hips)

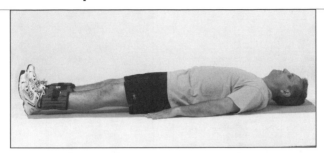

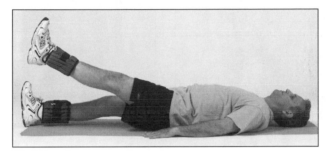

Lie on your back with your legs straight and your toes flexed. Your arms should be at the side of your body with their palms up. Now, lift one leg approximately 12 to 18 inches off the floor and hold for ten seconds. Lower the leg back down, but don't allow the heel to touch the floor. Repeat 10 times, then switch to other leg. Perform the recommended number of sets (I suggest 3) on each side.

Standing Knee Raise (Hip Flexion)

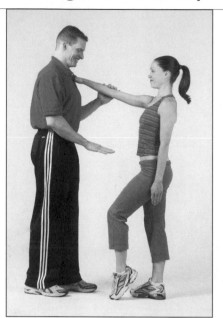 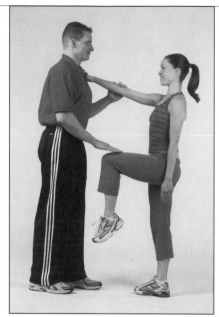

Start by standing next to a secure stationary object, arm's length away. Bend both of your knees slightly. Place one of your feet about six inches in front of the other. Point your toes down into the floor. Now, keeping your heel up, lift your leg up off the ground, knee first. Stop when your thigh is parallel to the floor. Remember never to go past a 90-degree angle at your knee joint. Lower your leg back to the starting position in a slow and controlled manner. Contact the floor with the toes of the working leg only; however, do not put your foot back down. Instead, immediately elevate your leg once more. You should try to maintain as much tension on the lifting leg as possible for the entire exercise. A variation of this exercise can be performed lying on your back.

Inner Thigh Stretch (Thighs)

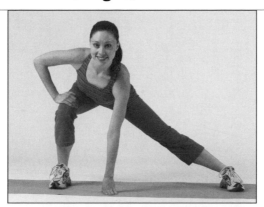

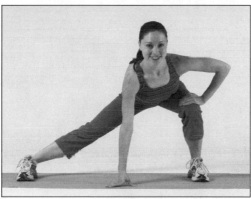

Lunge to the side with one leg, holding the position for several seconds, then repeat on the opposite side. To make this stretch more difficult, have your outstretched foot touch the floor with only your heel, and point your toes up.

Hip Flexor Stretch (Hip Flexors)

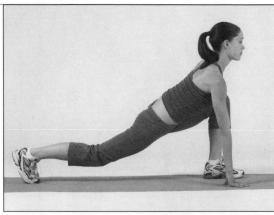

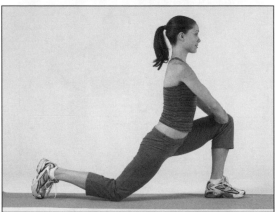

This alternate lower body stretch uses the lunge form to stretch the hip flexors. Lunge forward, resting your hand on your forward knee. Now drop your outstretched knee to the floor and raise your chest.

Seated Glute Stretch (Glutes)

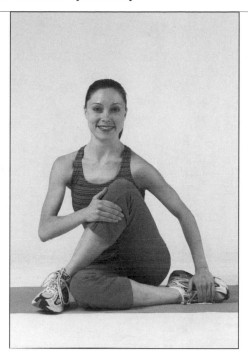

Sit on the floor with your knees bent and cross one leg over the other, as shown. Lean in toward your leg, keeping your head up. Repeat with the other leg.

Standing Glute Stretch (Glutes)

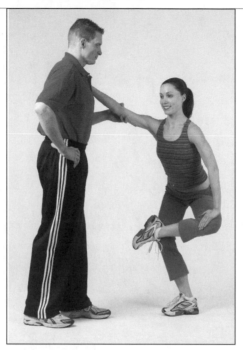

Place one ankle on a stationary object approximately hip height, or use a partner's support. Lean forward slightly. Repeat with the opposite leg.

Upper Body

There are five major muscle groups in the upper torso of the body: the Pectoral major (chest) latissimus dorsi (back), deltoids (shoulders), and the arms (biceps or front of the arms, triceps or back of the arms, and forearms or lower arms).

For some of these exercises, you will have the option to change hand positions from neutral (palms inward), to pronated (palms downward), to supinated (palms upward). This is for variety and it also alters the angle of resistance, keeping the muscles responsive over time. It is your choice to attempt three sets of one grip or just one set for each of the three different possible positions. Remember, during all variations be sure to concentrate on squeezing the scapulas (shoulder blades) together. (This is referring to several exercises in the Back section, notably the Low and High Pulls with Band.)

Push-Up on Knees (Chest)

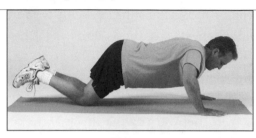

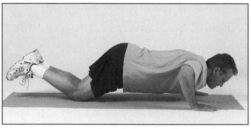

Begin by positioning your body on your hands and knees on an exercise mat on the floor. Place your hands shoulder width apart on the mat and at mid-chest level, not higher than your head or wider than your shoulders. Now lower your hips to the floor, making sure they are far enough back that your back can remain straight throughout the movement. Keep your head in line with your spine and your abdominals contracted. Now lower your torso until your elbows are at right angles. Do not go deeper; it may lead to shoulder injury. Extend from the elbows and hands to push back to the starting position. Do not lock out the elbow joints at any time.

Push-Up on Toes (Chest)

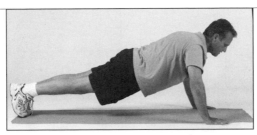

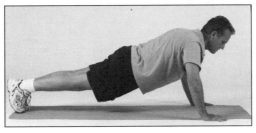

Start in a push-up position on your hands and toes. You should be in a plank position, not lying flat on the floor, as doing so will place stress on your shoulder and elbow joints. Your hands should be at mid-chest level. Keep your head in line with your spine and your abdominals contracted. Lower your torso to the ground until your elbow joints are at right angles. Extend from the elbows and hands to push back to the starting position. Do not lock out the elbow joins at anytime.

Bench Incline Push-Up (Chest)

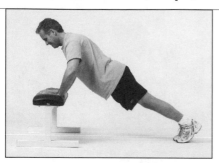 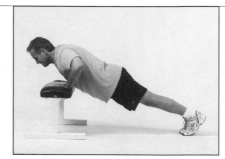

Performing this exercise on a bench changes the angle of resistance, but does not target a different muscle group. Position your torso directly over the bench with your hands shoulder width apart. Shift your weight slightly forward, so that you are resting on the balls of your feet. Keep your head in line with your spine and your abdominals contracted. Lower your body toward the bench until your elbows are at right angles and close to your torso. Push back away from the bench. Do not lock your elbow joints.

Bench Decline Push-Up (Chest)

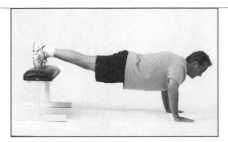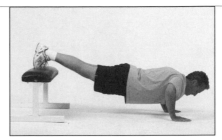

This variation places maximum tension on your chest, because of its inverted position and gravity. Because of this, it should be attempted only by the more advanced. Your hands should be shoulder width apart. Keep your head in line with your spine and your abdominals contracted in order to keep your back flat. Push up by extending your elbows, making sure to not lock them. Rest your feet on your toes throughout the exercise.

Wall Push-Up (Chest)

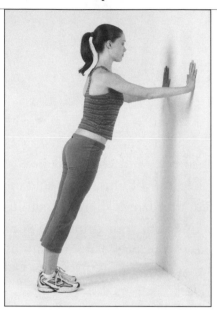
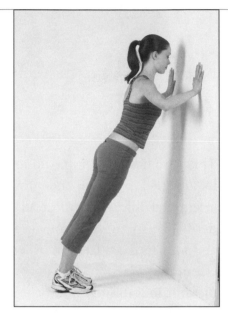

Stand facing a wall about an arm's length away. Now lean slightly forward to reach it, placing your hands on the wall at mid-chest level. Bend your elbows at right angles as your body moves closer to the wall. Stop before the angle becomes too great (more than 90 degrees). Hold your abdominals tight to help stabilize the torso. Extend your arms straight to push yourself back from the wall, being careful not to lock your elbow joints.

Flat Bench Dumbbell Press (Chest)

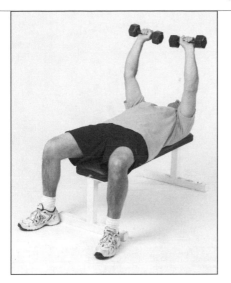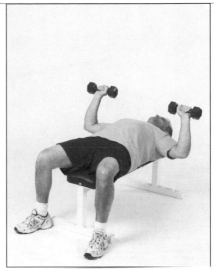

Lie on your back on a flat bench, a dumbbell in each hand. Extend your arms straight up over the middle of your chest, so that the dumbbells are touching. Start the movement by bending your elbows, lowering the dumbbells until your elbows reach a 90-degree angle. Do not go past this right angle position. Press the dumbbells up and together in one motion to return to the start position. Do not lock your elbows.

Flat Bench Press with Bodybar (Chest)

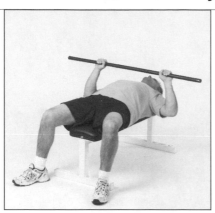 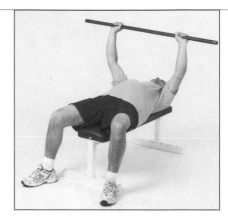

Lie on your back on a flat bench, grasping a bodybar with a grip slightly wider than shoulder width apart. Extend the bar directly over the midline of your pectoral muscles. Now lower the bar so your elbow joints create right angles. The bar should not make contact with the chest at any time. Press the bar back up to return to the start position. Do not lock your elbows.

Incline Bench Press with Bodybar (Chest)

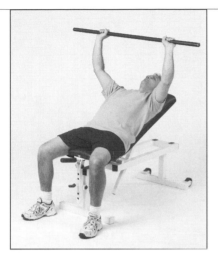 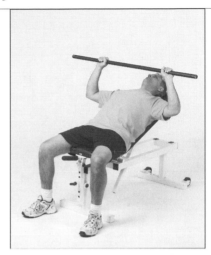

Lie down on an incline bench. Grip the bodybar slightly wider than shoulder width. Extend the bar straight up toward the ceiling, not directly over the head or out away from the body. Then lower the bar so that your elbows make a right angle. Do not lower the bar below your chin. Be careful to not to lock your elbows during the exercise.

Incline Bench Dumbbell Press (Chest)

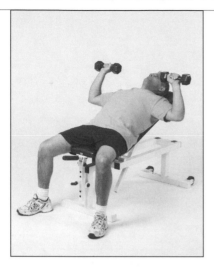 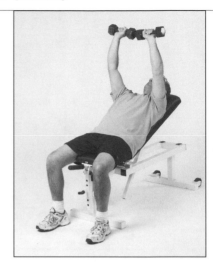

Incline the bench to no higher than 35 degrees (any higher will force you to engage your deltoids). Grasp one dumbbell in each hand with your palms facing away from you. To start, hold the dumbbells in fully extended arms over the midline of your chest. Depress your scapula, pressing your shoulder blades into the back of the bench. Bring the dumbbells down, bending your elbows. Do not drop your elbows below your body at the bottom, which would stress your shoulder joints, and be careful not to lock your elbow joints at the top of the movement.

By inclining the bench, you are changing the angle of resistance and forcing the pectoral muscles to adapt to a stress that is slightly different from a flat bench press or a push-up.

Flies with Band (Chest)

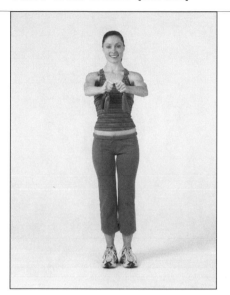 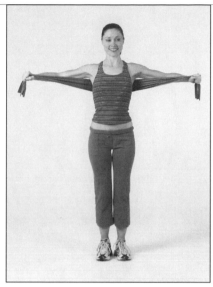

Stand with your back toward where the band is attached (a stationary object like a doorjamb). You can also wrap the band around your back as pictured. You may change the length of the band to increase or decrease the intensity of the exercise. Maintain proper posture during the entire exercise. Begin with your arms extended to the sides, elbows bent slightly, and hands level with the midline of your chest, palms facing forward. Extend your arms out away from your body, as if you were hugging a tree. Make sure you still have flexion in your elbow joint at the end of the movement. Do not lock your joints. Return to the starting position slowly, being careful not to extend past the right angle of the elbows.

Presses with Band (Chest)

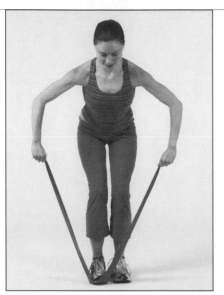 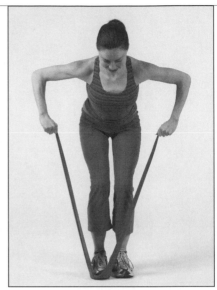

Stand with your feet together, stepping on the band. Begin with your arms extended out down towards your feet. Now bend your elbows so they make a right angle with your torso. Do not let your elbows go behind your body at any time. Do not lock your elbows.

Chest Stretch

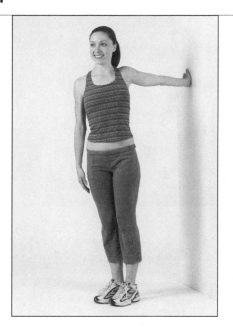

Grab a secure object at shoulder height with one hand. With your arm outstretched, turn away from the arm slightly (do not turn excessively). Hold the stretch for 15 seconds and repeat on the other side. Do not turn your shoulder in, bend your neck down, or hold the object too high.

Low Cable Row (Back)

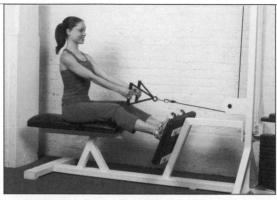

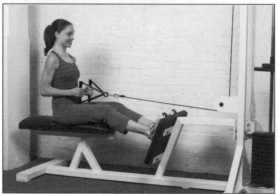

Sit on the floor or on the edge of a bench. You will be using a row machine. Place your feet on supports with your knees flexed and your back straight. Do not lean or be pulled forward by the weight. Pull the weight into your abdominals at your navel, making sure that your elbows are at right angles to your torso. Now stretch your arms back out to return to the starting position. Keep your head up and your abs tight at all times to help stabilize your spine. Don't bend forward at any point.

Reverse-Grip Lat Pulldown (Back)

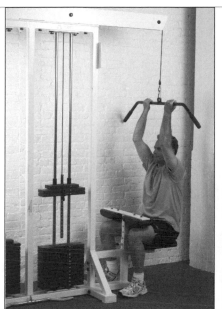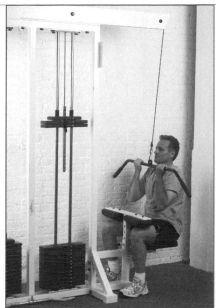

Sit with the pad above your thighs. You will be using a pulldown machine. You should hold the bar with a slightly wider than shoulder width undergrip. Make sure your back is straight and your abs are tight. Depress your scapulas, then pull the bar to chin level. Do not pull down or press down behind your head—this can cause injury to your shoulders. Do not lean back and pull to your chest, as doing so uses your biceps.

Lat Pulldown (Back)

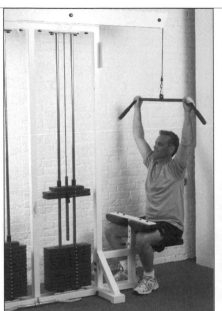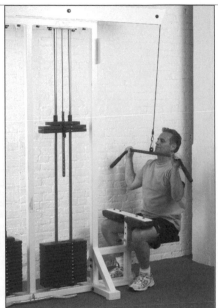

Place your hands on the bar slightly wider than shoulder-width apart, your palms facing away from your body. You will be using a pulldown machine. Pull down until the bar is at chin level. Going beyond this point can result in shoulder injury. Return the bar back overhead, making sure not to completely straighten your arm at the top of the movement.

Bent-Over Dumbbell Row (Back)

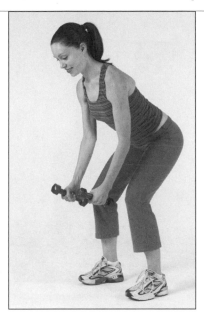 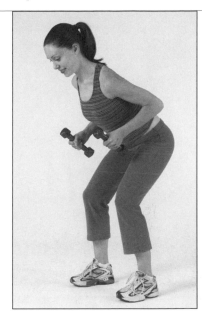

Bend over at the waist with a dumbbell in each hand. Contract the abdominals to support the lower back. If you have a lower back issue, perform the single arm variation instead. Allow the arms to hang straight down from the shoulder. Start by pulling the hands to the body, reaching a 90-degree right angle at the elbow joint. Stop when the dumbbells reach hip level. Keep your head up and your back straight.

Single Arm Dumbbell Row (Back)

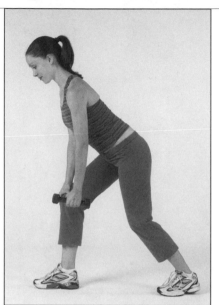
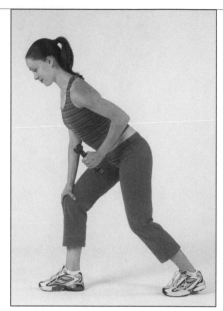

Hold a dumbbell in one hand and place the opposite hand on a stationary object or on your thigh, and step forward with one foot, as shown. Your weight should be evenly distributed among your legs and your supportive arm. Bring the dumbbell up toward your hip (do not bring it all the way up to your armpit). Keep your back flat and your head up.

High Pull with Band (Back)

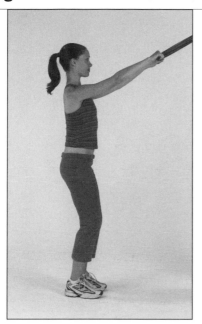 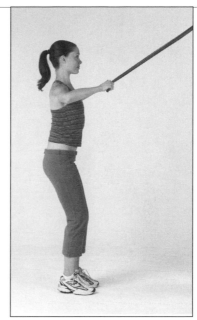

Attach a resistance band to a secure object or use a doorjamb accessory. Stand up straight with your knees partially bent. Place the band at a high position and pull back and down toward your body until your elbows are at right angles along the sides of your torso. Do not pull down too far. Be sure to keep your shoulder blades back and down during the entire exercise. Try squeezing them together slightly at the bottom of the motion. Return the arms back up to the starting position.

Low Pull with Band (Back)

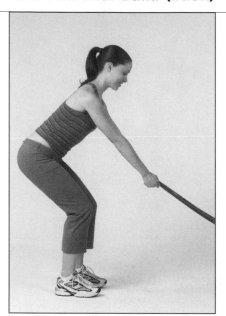 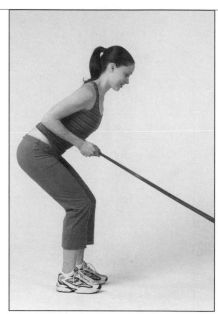

Start by attaching the band to a low position and bend over at the waist, making sure to keep your back straight and your abdominals contracted. Pull the band in to the body until your elbows are at right angles along the sides of your torso. Do not pull too far back. Allow your arms to extend outward away from the body in order to repeat the motion.

Lat Stretch

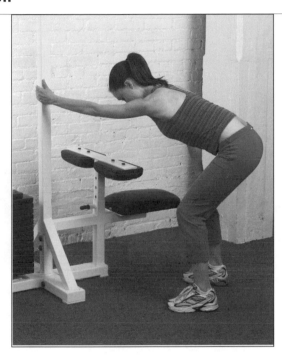

With your knees slightly bent and your back flat, grab a stationary object with one arm and pull back. Feel the stretch in your back. Hold for 15 seconds and repeat on the other side. Keep your head in line with your spine and do no lock your knees.

Standing Bodybar Press (Shoulders)

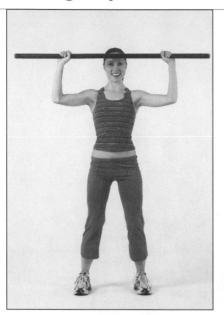 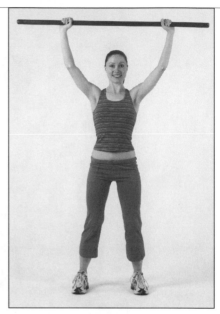

Use a bodybar instead of a barbell, as it is easier to control. Stand with your feet about shoulder width apart and tighten your abs to help stabilize the spine. Grip the bar with your hands slightly wider than shoulder width apart and use an overhand placement. Bring the bar up to chin level to begin the pressing movement. Extend your arms straight up toward the ceiling, making sure the bar is not out away from the body or behind the head. Stop before your elbows lock, pause, and then lower it back down until it reaches ear level. Be careful to not lower it too quickly so you always remain in control of the weight. For a variation, try this with dumbbells; however, be aware that controlling free weights is more difficult, so begin with lighter weights.

Dumbbell Lateral Raise (Shoulders)

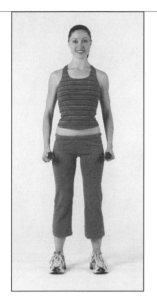 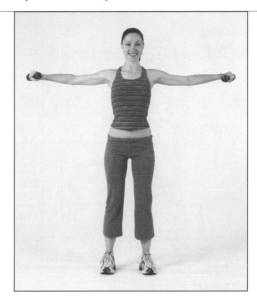

This is the most common incorrectly performed exercise. Stand straight with your feet shoulder width apart and knees slightly flexed. Hold the dumbbells in your hands with your palms face each other, elbows slightly bent, and arms at your sides. Raise your arms slowly up to the starting position, inhaling slowly. Keep a slight bend in your elbow throughout the entire range of motion. Do not raise the dumbbells over your shoulders, which will place stress on the shoulders and may injure your rotator cuff. Concentrate on extending your arms laterally before lifting them straight up.

Bent-Over Rear Delt Raise with Band (Shoulders)

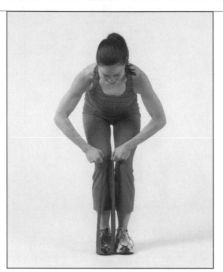 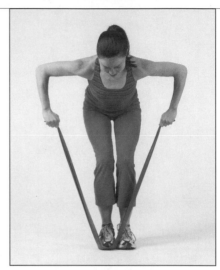

Begin by bending at the waist. Keep your back straight, your abdominals contracted, and your head level with your spine throughout the exercise. Hold the band at its ends, standing on it with one or both feet to create tension. To add resistance, spread your feet apart. Bend your elbows at a right angle, pulling the band out and upward. Be sure not to allow the arms to drop back or down, keeping them away from the sides of your body at all times. Try visualizing that strings are attached to your elbows and they are being pulled up toward the ceiling.

Seated Dumbbell Press (Shoulders)

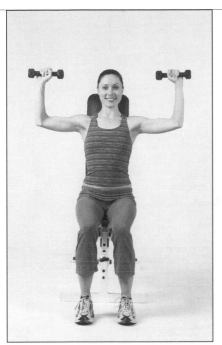 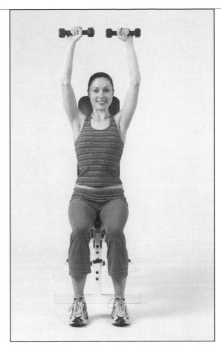

Sit on the bench with your feet flat on the floor. The bench doesn't need to be completely vertical, but it should support your lower back. Hold the dumbbells out to your sides at ear level and depress your scapulas. Raise the dumbbells overhead, being careful not to lock your elbows at the top. Keep the space between your ears and elbows as open as possible. Be sure to keep your elbows and hands completely vertical to avoid putting undue pressure on your joints.

Shoulder Stretch

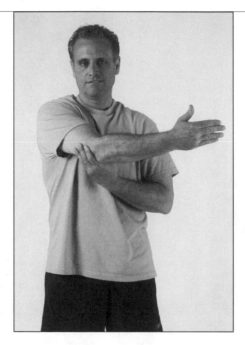

Hold one bent elbow with your opposite hand and pull it slightly across your body. Keep your shoulder relaxed. Hold for 15 seconds and repeat on the opposite side. Make sure to keep your neck in line with your spine. Your elbow should be pointing toward the ground, not in front of you.

Neck Stretch

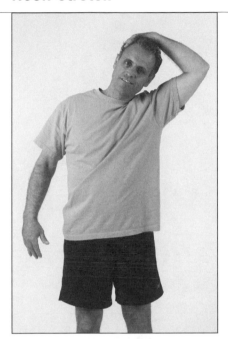 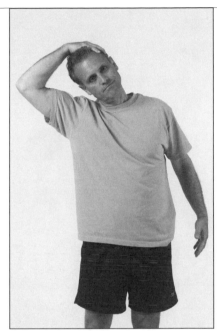

Place one hand on the opposite side of your head, and tilt your head to the side, as shown. Repeat on the opposite side. Then put both of your hands on the back of your head and bring your chin toward your chest. Do not tilt your head back—doing so can damage the cartilage in your neck.

Seated Dumbbell Curl (Biceps)

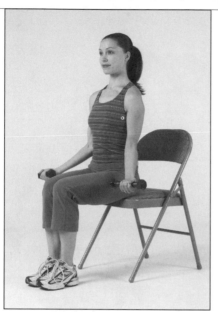 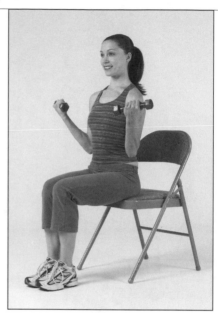

Sit on the end of a bench or chair, or stand with your feet together. Let your arms hang down along your sides. Begin the movement by bending your elbows. Raise your hands up and towards your shoulders, keeping the upper arm stationary. Your wrists should stay completely straight at all times. Pause the movement when the dumbbells reach shoulder height. Lower the dumbbells back down, making sure that the resistance is not swinging back and forth. The palms of the hands should be face up once clear of the legs.

Seated Alternating Dumbbell Curl (Biceps)

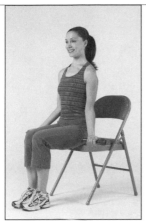 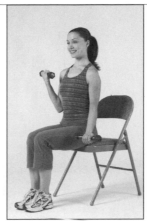 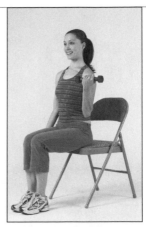

Sit on the edge of a chair or bench with your feet together, or stand. Let your arms hang down along your sides. Start the movement by bending the elbow of one arm, keeping the opposite arm still. Raise your hand up and toward the shoulder, keeping the upper arm stationary. Turn your wrist as your hand passes thigh level, so that at the top of the movement (at shoulder height) your hand is palm up. At the bottom of the movement your palms should face each other. Alternate arms. Make sure not to swing the weights when switching arms.

Standing Cable Curl (Biceps)

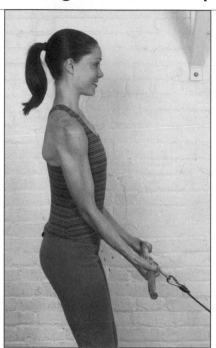 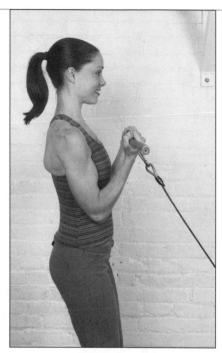

Keeping a slight bend in your knees, your back straight, and your abs tight, stand close to and parallel to the cable, with your elbows slightly in front of your body, not cocked in back of your body. Your hands should be shoulder width apart on the bar. As you curl the cable up, keep your wrists straight, not curled back. Concentrate on maintaining continuous tension in your biceps. The only moving joints should be the elbows; keep the rest of your body motionless. Raise the cable only to shoulder level, not to chin level.

Standing Bodybar Curl (Biceps)

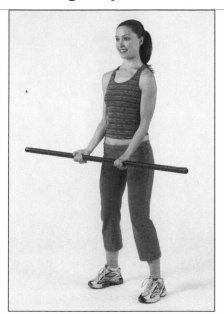 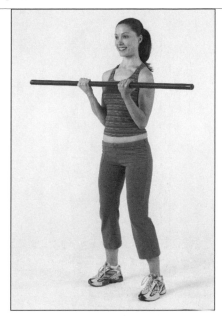

Stand straight with your feet shoulder width apart. Hold the body-bar in front of you with a slightly wider than shoulder width underhand grip. Lift the bar to shoulder level and slowly lower down again. Do not curl your wrists. Make sure to keep your back straight.

Hammer Curl (Biceps)

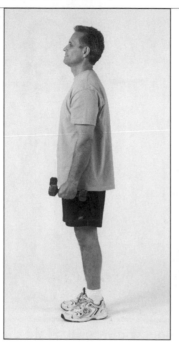 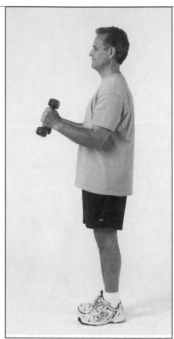

Stand, holding a dumbbell in each hand at your sides so that your palms face your legs. You should be holding them as you would hold a hammer. Raise the dumbbells only high enough for a 90-degree angle to form at your elbows, while maintaining the hammerlike grip.

Bicep Stretch

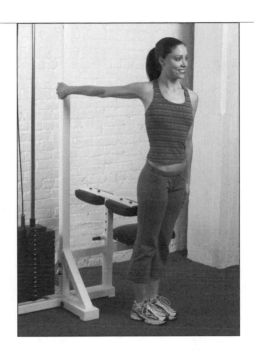

Grasp an object at shoulder height with your hand. Your grip should be reversed so that your thumb points down. With your arm outstretched, turn away from the arm slightly (do not turn excessively). Hold the stretch for 15 seconds and repeat on the other side. Do not turn your shoulder in, bend your neck down, or hold the object too high. All of these could be dangerous to the shoulder joint.

Overhead Dumbbell Extension (Tricep)

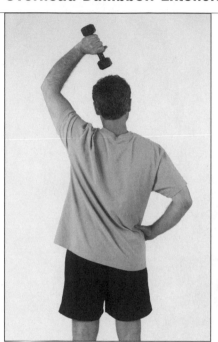 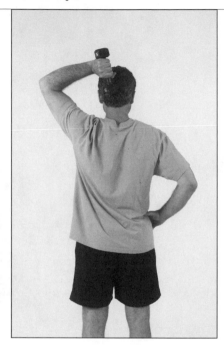

Stand with your knees slightly bent, your abs tight, back straight, scapula depressed, and one hand on your hip. With a dumbbell in the other hand, fully extend that arm over your head. Bend your elbow, bringing the dumbbell back behind your head. Keep your wrist straight. Repeat with the opposite arm.

Kickback (Tricep)

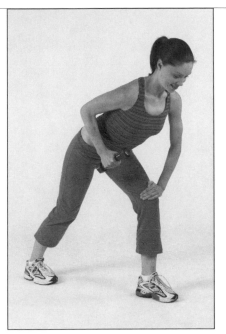 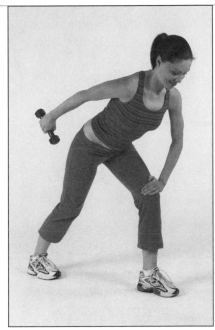

Step forward and put one hand on the forward knee to support your upper body. Hold a dumbbell in the other hand at your waist, then extend your arm straight back. Do not swing your arm back. Repeat with the other arm.

Triceps Pressdown (Triceps)

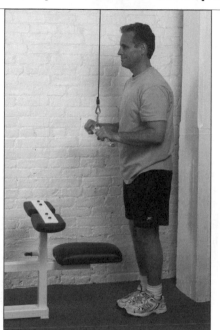 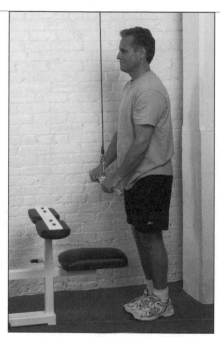

Stand facing a lat machine. Grasp a straight bar so that the palms are facing down towards the floor (overhand grip). Start with your arms at your sides and your elbows forming a 90-degree angle. Extend out and downward, with movement from the elbows only. Do not allow the upper arm to move back and forth at any time during the exercise. Maintain a straight wrist. Fully extend your elbow joint without locking out. Slowly return to the starting position.

Reverse Grip Pressdown (Triceps)

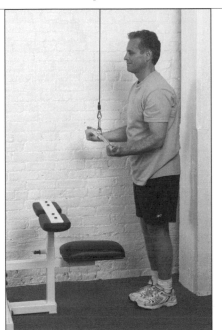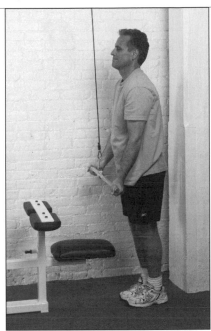

Stand facing a lat machine. Grasp a short curl bar attachment, with the palms facing up toward the ceiling (palms-up grip). Changing the grip position alters the angle, working the tricep muscle. Start with your upper arm stationary at the sides of your torso and your elbow joints at a 90-degree angle. Extend out and down, with movement from the elbows only. Keep your wrists straight throughout the exercise. Stop when fully extended at the elbow joints without locking. Slowly return to the starting position.

Rope Pressdown (Triceps)

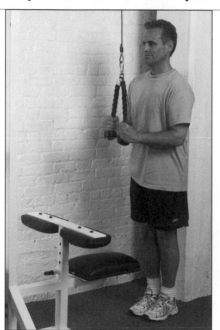 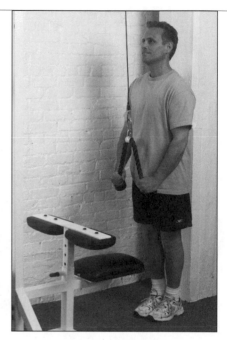

Stand facing a lat machine. Grasp a rope attachment so that your palms face each other. Take extra care to keep your wrists completely straight. Do not overgrip the rope. Start with a right angle in your elbow joints and your upper arms stationary along your sides. Extend out and down, allowing the hands to come apart slightly at the bottom of the movement. Do not pull too far with the hands, which would cause your wrists to bend excessively. Slowly return to the starting position.

Triceps Stretch

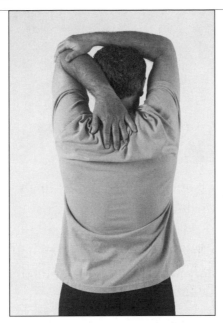

Grab one elbow behind your head with the opposite hand. Do not yank your body to the side. Hold and repeat on the opposite side.

Forearm Extension (Forearm)

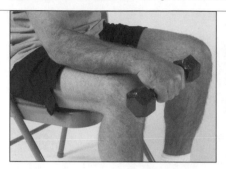 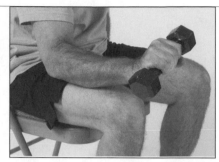

Sit on a chair. Place one forearm on your thigh. Grasp a dumbbell in one hand, your palm down. Relax the wrist so that it hangs over your knee. The knuckles should point toward the floor. The motion is small; pull only the hand back toward the body, not the arm. Be sure to keep your forearm in place on your thigh for entire exercise. Do not overgrip or squeeze the dumbbell.

Forearm Flexion (Forearm)

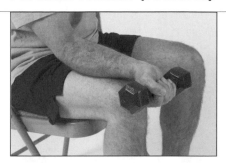 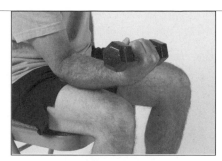

Sit on a chair. Place one forearm on your thigh. Hold a dumbbell with the palm up. Let the dumbbell relax in your hand and hang down toward your fingers. Curl the wrist up and toward the upper body. Make sure the forearm stays stationary on the thigh. Do not lift your arm up off your leg.

Forearm Rotation (Forearm)

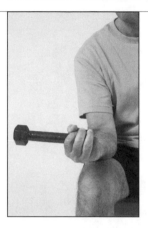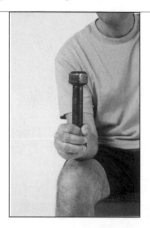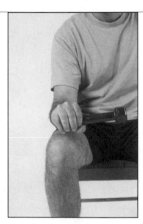

Sit on a chair. Place the forearm on your thigh. Hold one end of a dumbbell in your palm, the back of your wrist on your knee. The dumbbell should point to the outside. Rotate the dumbbell upward, so that the end now points straight up toward the ceiling. Continue rolling the wrist but keep the arm in place, not allowing your arm to slide back and forth over your thigh. Finish the movement by returning the dumbbell to the starting position.

9

A Positive Mental Approach

The mind-body connection is potentially the last place to discover new ways to excel at our physical abilities. If you have MS, this may sound intimidating because of the cognitive issues of the disease. It's sadly common that newly diagnosed MS patients think it is only a matter of time before they lose all control over their body and brain functions. While this is a very real fear, it's not accurate. The mind-body connection is well-documented in many different areas of medicine, sports, and wellness, but not yet with MS, as a majority of the medical community has chosen to focus on treating symptoms with drugs.

Even with all the advances in modern medical technology, there is so much that is still unknown or uncertain: from what causes someone to contract MS to the source of power behind the mind-body connection. What is known, however, is my personal experiences after six years of working with MS clients. Every single one of my clients possessed amazing determination, immeasurable in a traditional manner. The simple fact that we had the opportunity to work together proves that my clients had decided they were not going to settle for what was told to them.

A perfect example of this is my client Fran Rand. She is 71 years old, and she has been fighting MS for more than 20 years. For three years Fran trained with me religiously every week. She was one of the most consistent and dedicated clients I ever trained in my career. The only time that she missed a workout was when I had to cancel. She is just five feet tall and weighs maybe 100 pounds, but her internal strength is enormous. Her commitment not to let the disease dictate her life was truly an inspiration.

MS affected her left side, giving her a dropped foot and causing her to rely on a cane. She also had some general weakness on her left side, including her left arm and hand. We ended up using the cane in her training by strapping on one-pound Velcro ankle weights. I nicknamed this the "Fran Special" in her honor. As well as our weekly strength training workouts, she also attended aquatic classes twice a week. Her constant hard work paid off, and I believe it allowed her to remain active. Fran epitomized the "maintenance is progress" concept. It's never too late to begin exercising. Fran proved that every day.

With some, MS strikes them in the prime of their lives, which presents unique challenges. What do you do when your doctor tells you that you won't be able to do the things you enjoy doing without difficulty, and someday soon—maybe not at all? This can be overwhelming to accept for most individuals. Sometimes the doctor will prescribe antidepressants to help the newly diagnosed patient, but eventually you realize you aren't being given the answers you need, and so you seek out alternatives.

This was the case with one of my clients, a 31-year-old physical education teacher. She was always extremely active and in great shape at the time of her diagnosis, with no outwardly visible symptoms or specific loss of function. She did, however, have a lot of issues with fatigue and general weakness. For her, being told that she could not go "all out" was very hard to accept. Because of this, she was the perfect candidate for getting more from doing less, or maximum efficiency. Remember, with MS, you no longer have the luxury of being able to get away with more. More is just more of the same thing; it's not always better for your health.

Acceptance is a huge part of the equation when learning how to deal with MS. Another one of my clients, a very successful businessman and a competitive drag racer, kept his MS a secret for ten years. He made excuses for his lack of ability at crucial times. However, it wasn't until he faced the facts of his disease that he could come to terms with his new limitations, and from that point, he was able to learn how to create new abilities.

The brain is a muscle, and your mind can be trained just like the rest of your body. Do mental workouts several times a day by sitting in a quiet place and mentally taking your mind through your workout. Visualize yourself warming up, exercising your abdominals, and performing exercises in each muscle group with proper form and technique. Try to make your body mentally feel the physical changes you are experiencing, while completing every set in your mind's eye. This will be hard to make yourself do at first and it may seem silly, but try it and be consistent about doing these mental workouts just as much as the actual physical training, and you will be amazed how much it helps you achieve.

About the Model

The male model pictured is named Peter, and he has MS. He and I met for the first time the day of the photo shoot. He described his case as being pretty mild, and he had been diagnosed only two years prior, but he felt as if he had been fighting off MS for up to six years before the formal diagnosis. His primary problem is with his right leg and loss of strength in his quadriceps, and while he is not taking any medication for MS, he does have a workout routine he uses on a weekly basis.

When we began the photo shoot, I began to instruct him on proper form as well as safe ways to train effectively (smarter, not harder). As we continued to take photos, he struggled to finish, but I could see how much he was learning. By the end of the day he said he could see how being able to train smarter was going to have a huge effect in his workouts in the future. This occurred after just one day with someone I had never worked with before. Think of the possibilities this workout gives to you, the reader.

Part III: The Workouts

The Good Days and the Bad Days

If you ask people with MS how they are doing, they will answer by saying either it's a good day or it's a bad day. That's how life is with MS. On a good day, you can go out and do whatever you want to do (shop, do chores, work, or even exercise). On bad days, it feels as if just getting out of bed is impossible, and the fatigue by the end of the day can be overwhelming.

I experienced this with my clients firsthand, and what kind of day it was would determine how we would train. When they felt good, we would take advantage of their high energy levels. On the bad days, we modified the workout to fit.

It's important to mention that it's hard to assess your own physical limitations accurately. To help you determine if you're up for a Good Day workout or a Bad Day workout, don't make the decision until you have performed a proper warm-up and are a few exercises into the workout. You should learn how to read the messages your body is sending. A quick tip is to review the activities you have been involved in the 24 to 48 hours preceding your workout session. If you used a lot of energy recently, you may not be up for a vigorous workout.

Your body can handle only a limited amount of stress before that stress becomes detrimental to your health. Life, work, school, relationships, finances—all take a toll on your ability to cope. Exercise is a stressor on the body as well; however, it should relieve, not add, to your stress. MS is yet another source of stress, making it paramount for you to design exercises for your body. Learn to work within your body's natural range of motion to make sure you do not force your muscles to do something they cannot.

More exercise is not necessarily better exercise. Your body naturally adapts to repetitive movements, requiring you to do even more to get less. Because of this, it's best to teach your body by exercising at maximum efficiency. This is even more imperative for those with

MS, because you cannot afford to waste energy. The fatigue factor, as you well know, will kick in when your body simply cannot do any more. MS will eventually force you to stop. You can get around this by exercising on a regular schedule and developing an ability to cope with physical fluctuations. Once you learn how to get more by doing less, you'll receive the maximum benefits for energy spent.

You will accomplish this by creating a workout program based on the natural functions of your muscles, range of motion, and functionality. In other words, you will stick to the basics.

What Is a Bad Day Workout?

It's now possible to successfully train whether you are having a good or bad day. You will simply modify your workout. Not so surprisingly, it's when you test your physical limitations that you discover possibilities for greater capacity. Your bad days become an opportunity to uncover hidden physical abilities. My clients often say, "There's a lot more to this then I thought before coming to working out."

The largest difference between the Good and Bad Day workouts is the approach you take once you determine what kind of day it is. A Bad Day session does not necessarily mean that it will be of less value. On the contrary, these workouts can be of the greatest value to your overall progress because you went ahead and exercised regardless of your lessened physical ability. Because you stayed on course, this consistency will pay off.

You will soon enter a time of physical and personal discovery. Each day will present unique challenges. My advice to you is to do your best possible and move on to the next day for the next opportunity to continue your workouts. This program allows for a certain amount of flexibility, but you must remain disciplined. Don't make excuses for yourself, and avoid any possible distractions that could keep you from your goals. For hints, see Chapter Nine, "A Positive Mental Approach."

The Workout

The Warm-up

You should warm up properly before you exercise. Be careful to warm up correctly, as there are many misconceptions about what this entails.

Do not stretch only before training. This only places tension upon muscles that are not yet ready. What's known as the traditional method of stretching can actually lead to injury. Remember, your muscles are like rubber bands. Before you warm up your muscles, they react as if they were frozen. In other words, if moved too much or too soon, your muscles can be strained, pulled, or torn.

To warm up safely, think once more about the frozen rubber band. You would thaw the band before using it by increasing the temperature of the rubber band itself, perhaps by putting it into a cup of hot water. It's the same for your muscles. To warm up, you must raise the core temperature of your body, or injury can occur. Simply holding static stretches will not achieve this.

Instead, you should perform low-intensity cardiovascular exercises, such as riding a stationary bike or walking on a treadmill, for five to ten minutes. At this point you should begin your stretches. By warming up properly, you are assisting in your own injury prevention.

The Total-Body Approach

The actual workout itself is a total-body approach. This routine will cover every muscle group by working just one exercise per group. To those who have tried other workout programs, this may sound strange, but it is surprisingly effective. If a muscle has only one function or range of motion, then only one exercise for that function is needed. Persons who work out a single body part using several different exercises are wasting their time and energy.

In your workout, you will select one exercise for each major muscle group. Every time you return for a workout, you will select a different exercise. This variety will keep your body from adapting to your workouts. The order of workout will be larger muscles first, descending to the smallest muscles. This is so you train the largest groups to exhaustion without being limited by your weaker muscle groups. For example, if you had trained your biceps before your back, the biceps would fail long before your back muscles had been worked to completion. The proper order:

Warm-up (5 to 10 minutes)
Abdominals (20 to 30)
Quadriceps (20 to 30, each leg)
Hamstrings (20 to 30, each leg)
Calves (20 to 30, each leg)
Hips/ankles (20 to 30, each leg)
Chest (20 to 30)
Back (20 to 30)
Shoulders (20 to 30)
Biceps (20 to 30, each arm)
Triceps (20 to 30, each arm)
Forearms (20 to 30, each arm)

This total body workout is meant to be accomplished every other day, because you should not strength train any muscle group two days in a row. Muscles need 24 to 48 hours between sessions to allow them to rest properly. If this rest period does not occur, the potential for injury dramatically increases. However, cardiovascular (aerobic) exercise can be performed daily.

Pacing for Good Days and Bad Days
You will be pacing yourself as you work out so you have the energy required to complete the exercises. To do this, you will be resting after each and every set. On good days, this rest may be only 30 to 45 seconds. On bad days, you may be required to take longer breaks, up to 1 to 2 minutes between sets. You can also use the time between sets to stretch the body part you are training.

There will be days when resting between sets simply isn't enough. In this situation, use the work-rest-pause method. Break the workout into two or more parts, taking an extended break between sections. During this break, engage in active recuperation, work on your walking technique, and then pick back up where you left off. There will be days when you are forced to stop completely. That's okay.

You should never go to a point where you are in pain. "No pain, no gain" is an out dated mind-set with no scientific merit and is responsible for many injuries.

Conclusion:
You Inspire Me

My fitness career has spanned more than twenty years and count-less clients. Nothing has been so challenging and personally reward-ing as working with those with MS. To give my clients what I felt they deserved—the possibility of an active life with MS—I was required to teach myself new skills so I could help to fight the dis-ease. It was only after the fact did I realize that I had learned as much from my clients as they had learned from me. I was truly inspired by every one of my MS clients, and I hope that the work we accomplished together will last as long as their impact on me has.

Thank you all.

Brad Hamler

Appendix A: Glossary

Acquired immune system: Allows the body to identify foreign cells, such as viruses, bacteria, and fungi, and differentiate them from its own cells. It also has the ability to remember foreign cells, so that it will automatically attack them if they reappear at another time.

Antigens: Protein molecules (although they can also be carbohydrates, DNA, and ribonucleic acid molecules) that provoke an immunological response from the body. They act as markers or identification tags attached to pathogens that invade and attack the body.

Auto-antigens: Antigens actually found in the body. They provoke an immunological response from the body against itself. One form of this response is called multiple sclerosis.

Axons: Long extensions that carry nerve transmissions along the length of the neuron. Unlike the dendrites, axons carry signals away from the soma. These electrochemical signals consist of a depolarizing current called an action potential. The axon is wrapped in the myelin, which insulates it as well as assists in the transmission of signals. However, myelin does not completely sheath the axon. It is broken up by junctions called nodes of Ranvier.

Blood-brain barrier: The cells lining blood vessels. The BBB's job is to allow oxygen, nutrients, carbon dioxide and other waste to flow between the blood and the central nervous system while blocking pathogens from getting into the brain. Immune system cells enter and attack the CNS of those with MS while they do not penetrate those without MS. This suggests that the BBB has become damaged, perhaps by a pathogen, and is no longer doing its job. Another theory is that a trauma, such as a fall or car accident, can damage the BBB, thus leading to the onset of MS.

Central and peripheral nervous systems: MS affects mainly the central nervous system (CNS), which is the brain and the spinal cord. Gray matter and white matter are the two regions that make up the CNS. Gray matter does all the processing, and white matter communicates between areas of gray matter and between gray matter and the rest of the body. The CNS contrasts with the peripheral nervous system, which is made up of nerves that transmit signals between the CNS and the rest of the body. The CNS contains billions of nerves cells called neurons, which facilitate thought processing, and trillions of glial cells, which help the CNS function by repairing damage and isolating it from the rest of the body. Although the lesions that initiate an MS attack affect primarily the white matter, they are found on gray matter 5% of the time.

Chemokines: A subset of cytokines. They attract white blood cells to the site of an infection.

Cytokines: Small proteins comprising just one amino acid strand; they modify the behavior of surrounding cells. Cytokines' main roles include cell activation, inflammatory tissue breakdown and repair, and the sending of signals directing certain cells to die.

Dendrites: Thin branchlike extensions that exchange signals with other neurons across a connection called a synapse. The synapse sends electrochemical signals or neurotransmitters across the synapse cleft, which is the gap between neurons. Dendrites carry these signals toward the soma, or the main body of the neuron.

DNA: A double-stranded helix, the building blocks of genes. DNA resembles a rope ladder and holds chemical codes that manufacture cellular chemicals. DNA is also able to replicate itself.

Genes: Thought to play a major role in the onset and development of MS. Coupled with environmental factors, they determine the appearance, constitution, and behavior of all life on Earth. Most inherited traits are the result of two genes, one dominant and one recessive. The dominant gene is the one that manifests itself and may play a significant role in who and who doesn't develop MS. Every cell contains tightly wound ropes of genetic material called chromosomes.

Glial cells: Maintain and support the neurons of the CNS. Their duties include repair of damaged myelin and the production of scar tissue. The hairlike filaments of the glial cells hold neurons in place and keep their structure intact. Glial cells also produce potassium and calcium and regulate the level of neurotransmitters. Additionally, they clean the CNS by removing dead cells and other debris.

Immune system: Defends the body against pathogens, such as bacteria, viruses, and fungi, which can do harm to and even kill the patient. The immune system is actually two systems—the innate or natural immune system and the acquired or specific immune system.

Innate immune system: Consists of the skin, the inner walls of blood vessels, mucous layers, and other membranes, which act as barriers against invading pathogens. It also includes enzymes in the mucous and antibacterial proteins. Fever, a process in which the body overheats in order to kill invaders, is another important element of the innate immune system, as is inflammation, which counters threats by producing toxic chemicals such as nitrous oxide, hydrogen peroxide, and histamines. Finally, white blood cells, or leukocytes, actually devour invading pathogens. The innate immune system is unable to detect pathogens that have changed form in an attempt to evade detection and penetrate it.

Myelin: Produced by cells called oligodendrocytes, myelin is the smooth, fatty protein sheath protecting the neuron's axon. MS detroys not only the myelin of the CNS's white matter but also the oligodendrocyte and even the axon itself.

Neurons: Neurons or nerve cells are referred to as the body's "controlling cells." They are generally believed to be the most important cells in the nervous system. Their job is to think, to memorize, to control both conscious and unconscious bodily functions, to process sensory stimulation, and to transmit voluntary and involuntary movement and signals to and from all parts of the body.

Oligodendrocytes: A type of glial cell; they produce the fatty protein called myelin, which insulates the axon portion of the neuron. Each oligodendrocyte produces myelin for several axons, and each axon can be supplied by several oligodendrocytes, which wrap around the axons in thin, paperlike sheets. As oligodendrocytes attempt to replace myelin destroyed by MS, they are often themselves destroyed, hindering the repair process and making the symptoms of the disease even worse.

Appendix B:
Training Log

Bad Day/Good Day: _____

Date: _____

Starting Time: _____

Ending Time: _____

EXERCISES CHOSEN

Abdominals: _____

Quadriceps: _____

Hamstrings: _____

Calves: _____

Hips/Ankles: _____

Chest: _____

Back: _____

Shoulders: _____

Biceps: _____

Triceps: _____

Forearms: _____

Walking Exercises: _____

NOTES:

_____

_____

Appendix C:
Resources

ADA Home Page

Information and technical assistance on the Americans with
Disabilities Act.
www.usdoj.gov/crt/ada

CLAMS: Computer Literate Advocates for Multiple Sclerosis

Computer information and communication for people with MS, by
people with MS.
www.clams.org

NARIC: The National Rehabilitation Information Center

Visitors can submit requests, search database, read RehabWire, explore
research from the National Institute on Disability and Rehabilitation,
and more.
www.naric.com

National Multiple Sclerosis Society

A nonprofit organization serving patients with multiple sclerosis in
United States by supporting scientific research.
www.nationalmssociety.org

MSWorld

MSWorld™, the National MS Society's collaborative partner, contains
the official chat and message board site for persons with MS.
www.msworld.org/communications.htm